Dementia

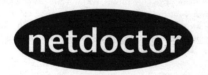

Series Editor
Dr Dan Rutherford
www.netdoctor.co.uk

Copyright © 2004 by NetDoctor.co.uk
Illustrations (except figure 5) copyright © 2004 by Amanda Williams

First published in Great Britain in 2004

The right of NetDoctor.co.uk to be identified as the Author
of the Work has been asserted by them in accordance
with the Copyright, Designs and Patents Act 1988.

10 9 8 7 6 5 4 3 2 1

British Library Cataloguing in Publication Data
A record for this book is available from the British Library

ISBN 0 340 86267 X

Typeset in Garamond by Avon DataSet Ltd,
Bidford-on-Avon, Warwickshire

Printed and bound in Great Britain by
Bookmarque Ltd, Croydon, Surrey

The paper and board used in this paperback are natural recyclable
products made from wood grown in sustainable forests.
The manufacturing processes conform to the environmental
regulations of the country of origin.

Hodder & Stoughton
A Division of Hodder Headline Ltd
338 Euston Road
London NW1 3BH
www.madaboutbooks.com

Contents

Foreword   ix
Acknowledgements   xi

1   **General aspects of dementia**   1
    What is dementia?   1
    Dementia treatment and care   2
    Types of dementia   3
    Features of Alzheimer's disease   4
    Time scale   6
    Dementia in practice   7
    Formal systems of disease description   8

2   **The brain, ageing and dementia**   9
    Brain facts   9
    Confusion and dementia   10
    Brain structure   10
    Nerve signalling   12
    Neurotransmitters   14
    Computers and brains   14
    Adaptability of nerve connections   15
    Normal ageing   16
    Changes seen in dementia   17
    Establishing the type of dementia   19

3   **The causes of dementia**   20
    Alzheimer's disease   20
    Vascular disease   23
    Strokes and dementia   27
    Causes of other types of dementia   28
    Protection against dementia   29
    More research needed!   33
    Taking the global view   34

4   Dementia diagnosis: (1) Symptoms and other   35
    considerations
    Memory loss   36
    Language problems   36
    Difficulties with the tasks of daily living   37
    Behaviour changes   37
    Mood   39
    Depression in the elderly   40
    Involving the patient   43

5   Dementia diagnosis: (2) Tests   44
    Assessing intellectual function   44
    MMSE   45
    Other mental function tests   46
    Use of tests of mental function   46
    Specialist referral   47
    Memory clinics   48
    Assessment process   49
    Confirming the diagnosis   50
    Specialised tests   51
    Test for a reason   52
    Informing the patient and the carers   52
    Advising on treatment   53
    Co-ordinating care   53
    Follow-up   53
    Present dementia care arrangements   54

6   Treatments for dementia   55
    Drug treatments   55
    Neurotransmitters and drug action   55
    Cholinesterase inhibitors   56
    Research trials in dementia   57
    Results of cholinesterase inhibitor drugs in dementia   58
    Memantine (Ebixa®)   60
    Vascular dementia   61
    Gingko biloba   61
    Drugs with uncertain or no proven benefit   62

Non-drug treatments   62
Other help   67

7   General principles of dementia care   69
Maintain dignity   69
Keep things normal   70
Avoid confrontation   70
Plan ahead   70
Keep it simple   71
Keep it safe   71
Keep healthy   71
Keep communicating   71
Memory aids   72
Relax   72
Be prepared to experiment   72

8   Behavioural problems in dementia   73
Depression   73
Agitation and aggression   74
Sleep disturbance   76
Wandering   76
Delusions and hallucinations   77

9   Caring for the carers   78
Emotions   78
Get help early   80
Look after yourself   80

Appendix A: References   82
Appendix B: Drugs   88
Appendix C: Useful contacts and addresses   95

Foreword

As we get older our memory is not as good as when we were young, although we all pride ourselves on our ability to remember events from our childhood or young adulthood. For some people, however, the loss of memory is not 'just your age'.

Dementia is a term used to describe the loss of intellectual, social and day-to-day functioning which affects a minority of people in old age. For those affected the consequences can be devastating. There are major effects on family life as the care needs of a person with dementia increase and in turn the carer too needs help and support.

This book identifies the main causes of dementia and briefly touches on the changes in the brain which lead to symptoms appearing. Symptoms are described in a clear and understandable way and importantly readers are helped to consider other problems which may mimic dementia or occur alongside dementia, making the person worse than they should be.

In the last seven or eight years the ability to treat dementia has improved with the advent of a new class of medication called cholinesterase inhibitors. The book gives a balanced approach to what might be expected from treatment with cholinesterase inhibitors, correctly recognising that the long-term benefits for carers or for the prevention of admission to institutional care remains uncertain. The treatment of problems which are not helped by these drugs is addressed and there is an examination of the effect of non-drug treatments, though often these are not as beneficial as sometimes thought.

Importantly, the book addresses the general principles of dealing with a person with dementia and their carer. For many years the principles outlined in these chapters were the mainstay of intervention and it is important that these are not lost with the advent of new drugs.

This book will be helpful to people who are concerned about their memory, to people with early dementia, to those who are involved in the day-to-day caring of people with dementia, or to those who are uncertain about what to do when they meet someone with dementia. Recognition of the illness at an early stage is crucial if the effects of treatment are to be maximised and if care needs are to be anticipated without crises occurring. More knowledge and understanding helps to prevent carers becoming isolated. This book should help increase knowledge of the condition and its recognition. I hope that it will be widely read.

Dr Peter Connelly, MB, ChB, FRCPsych
Consultant Old Age Psychiatrist
Murray Royal Hospital
Perth
Scotland

Acknowledgements

I am particularly grateful to Dr Peter Connelly, Consultant in Old Age Psychiatry at Murray Royal Hospital, Perth, who kindly reviewed this book in detail and made many helpful suggestions despite the considerable other demands on his time.

Lesley Beresford from the North Cornwall Community Mental Health Team sent me details of the shared care pathway for people with dementia that has been developed in that part of the country and which was an excellent reference source.

Julie, Patrick and Amanda at Hodder have as always been completely supportive in helping me to add another title to this series, as have Anne and David at home.

Although great care is taken to ensure that the information presented here is accurate, there is always a chance that errors have crept in. Please let me know if you spot any or if you have any suggestions for ways in which this or any other book in the series could be improved. I can be contacted at d.rutherford@netdoctor.co.uk by putting 'Hodder' in the subject line.

Dr Dan Rutherford BSc, MB, ChB, MRCGP, FRCP(Edin)
Medical Director
www.netdoctor.co.uk

Chapter 1

General aspects of dementia

What is dementia?

Dementia can be very briefly defined as a slowly progressive impairment of a person's intellectual and social functions. It usually results in loss of memory as well as of the ability to make decisions, to carry out day-to-day tasks like using the phone or managing money, and to think in abstract ways. Someone with dementia may appear perplexed and may also show changes in their personality and behaviour. Although one can generalise on many of the features of dementia, as we do in this book in trying to describe the condition, in practical terms dementia is very much an individual illness. The degrees by which an affected person's various mental abilities are impaired vary between individuals and can fluctuate over time. Someone's background educational level, their level of social support, the state of their mental and physical health in other respects and whether they are on medication for other reasons all have a bearing on the impact of dementia. Against such a background one can see that brief descriptions of dementia are by necessity rather inadequate.

Dementia treatment and care

Had this book been written even ten years ago it would not have been very encouraging to read. Dementia is a condition that gets worse with time and until fairly recently there was not a lot one could do about it. We are still a long way from having cures, as will become clear later, but the treatments now available can slow the onset of some symptoms of dementia. Research into dementia is intensive and we can hope to see advances in treatment over the next few years.

PRESENT AND FUTURE TRENDS

With the many improvements in the general care of the elderly that have occurred in recent years, many people with mild to moderate dementia now survive for decades. The increased survival of older people who have long-term illnesses like dementia has, however, increased the load on health and social services, and this is set to become even more pronounced with the increase in numbers of affected people in the community.

According to the Alzheimer's Society and the government's National Service Framework for Older People dementia currently affects over 775,000 people in the UK. This equates to more than 5 per cent of the population aged 65 and over and 20 per cent of the population aged 80 and over. Dementia can also affect people in younger age groups; it is estimated there are currently 17,000 people with the condition who are under 65 years old and 154,000 people with dementia currently live alone. The Alzheimer's Society projections are that by 2010 there will be 840,000 people with dementia in the UK and by 2050, 1.5 million.

The annual cost to the health service of dementia care currently exceeds £6 billion.

CARE ARRANGEMENTS

The ways in which we care for people with dementia are changing, driven in part by the pressure of increasing numbers, but also by changing values within medicine and society. As recently as the 1980s people with severe dementia were housed in long-term psychiatric hospitals. Such units are far less common and in their place is a mixture of care-in-the-community support or private residential and nursing home placements. Simultaneously medical expertise in the care of dementia has expanded and many parts of the country are well served by multidisciplinary teams of experts from all the relevant health and social services, who pull together and ensure the best care is delivered to those clients referred to them.

The legacy of the many politically driven changes to the NHS of the 1980s and 1990s has, however, left us with a patchwork of dementia care in the UK. Some areas are well served whereas others are inadequately resourced or set up. The quality of care delivered to people with dementia in the UK is on average high but is often too dependent on the personal input of overworked members of the primary care team.

Types of dementia

Dementia is diagnosed primarily on the basis of the symptoms and effects it has on a person's function. Doctors refer to it as a 'clinically diagnosed' condition, meaning that once a careful history and examination has been undertaken by the doctor, including listening to the observations of relatives or carers as needed, it will then usually be possible to diagnose it. Medical tests do have an important role, but mainly to exclude the presence of other conditions that might mimic dementia or which are important if

3

they exist alongside dementia (such as, for example, poor circulation or diabetes).

'Dementia' is actually an umbrella term for a group of illnesses with similar effects. There are three main types of dementia:

1 Alzheimer's disease
2 Vascular dementia
3 Dementia with Lewy bodies

'Mixtures' of these types of dementia are common, especially in people over 80. They are all described in more detail in chapter 2. Of these, Alzheimer's disease is the most common, indeed people commonly take 'Alzheimer's disease' to be an alternative general term for 'dementia'. Although this is incorrect it is useful to list the features of Alzheimer's disease because they are typical of all forms of dementia.

Features of Alzheimer's disease

MEMORY LOSS

Memory loss usually occurs early in dementia. Recall of recent events (short-term memory) is usually affected more prominently than recall for events further in the past (long-term memory), although both are affected to some degree. It is as if the normal process we have of shifting new information and experiences into our memory store is disrupted, and new memories do not get filed away in a fashion in which they can be accessed appropriately.

Forgetfulness is of course something we all experience and it tends to be more noticeable with ageing. The distinctions between the early stages of dementia and the normal effects of ageing on the brain are not clear-cut. Often it is only the passage of time and the progression of memory loss and other symptoms that make it possible to diagnose dementia. Increasing public awareness of dementia is a good thing but it can cause anxiety about the future in someone whose memory begins to fail a bit. Most people who experience this will not in fact go on to develop dementia. Equally, someone who is beginning to develop dementia may notice memory loss as the first sign of the illness, and this can cause worry and depression over how the illness may later progress.

Difficulties in learning new tasks are a prominent feature of dementia and reflect the problems with memory storage. The ability to perform previously well-learned activities is often preserved for longer. As time goes by the other features below appear, although not in any typical order.

LANGUAGE DIFFICULTY

Examples are difficulty in finding the right word, causing hesitation or the substitution of a wrong word (calling a plate a cup perhaps). Other ways in which this may show are word repetition, stammering, the failure to complete sentences or losing the train of thought during speech. The medical term for this problem is 'aphasia'.

IMPAIRED ABILITY TO CARRY OUT 'MOTOR' ACTIVITIES

Motor activities are any actions requiring the use of voluntary muscles. Making a cup of tea, writing a letter or walking about require a range of high-speed mental processing and muscle co-ordination, operating at both the conscious and subconscious levels, which we normally take for granted. We have to be aware of where our body, limbs and hands are at any given moment, where we want them to go next, how fast to do so and with what purpose, what to do once the action is finished and so on. One has to be careful here to ensure that any observed difficulties are not due to a physical impairment, such as for example the effect of a previous stroke. 'Apraxia', to give it its medical term, is the inability to carry out motor activity despite intact muscles and nerves. It can show up in any practical task but common areas of trouble are dressing, feeding, bathing and other activities of self-care.

DIFFICULTY IN RECOGNISING OR IDENTIFYING OBJECTS

To give a name to a person, object, sound or smell, or otherwise make sense of the input we receive from our senses, requires us to analyse the incoming information and then compare it with our store of knowledge. If there is a match then we can identify the object or sensation. Again this is something normally done subconsciously and at high speed. 'Agnosia' is the medical term for problems such as this occurring in the absence of impairment of the senses themselves.

IMPAIRED 'EXECUTIVE FUNCTION'

This is a jargon term for planning and organising things. Executive function often requires some degree of abstract thinking as well as the ability to put things in their right order to make them happen and refers to any task, no matter how basic or complex. Making a cup of tea requires that the water is first boiled and, prior to that, for the kettle to be filled with water, plugged in and switched on. All these actions need to be in the right order to achieve success. In dementia this process can go wrong at any point along the way.

Time scale

The natural behaviour of dementia is that it develops slowly, usually over several years. Rapid changes of someone's functional ability are more likely to be due to some other condition, some of which are noted later. This is not to say that events cannot move quickly in dementia. A common situation is for someone, perhaps with quite significant dementia, but who is managing to exist at home, to then develop some other problem that they cannot cope with. Often the problem that tips the balance is a medical one, such as a fall or a urine infection. Suddenly the precariously balanced home situation becomes unstable and a crisis develops. In some people with dementia this may be how they come for the first time to the attention of medical or social services. If they are resistant to help being offered from family, friends or carers yet are not in a position to adequately care for themselves, then such a situation can be very difficult to deal with.

Dementia in practice

Two people with dementia may share the same diagnosis but would still be quite different from each other. The exact pattern of dementia differs from person to person and the impact that dementia has is even more variable, as there are so many factors in someone's environment and social circumstances that matter.

Although it is useful to analyse and name all these individual ways in which brain function is affected in dementia this is not of course how they appear in life; in reality they are all mixed together. Some of the tests doctors use in diagnosing dementia are designed to assess these separate aspects of brain function and are covered in more detail in chapter 5.

Other medical conditions can cause some of the same problems that are seen in dementia. A stroke is an event caused usually by blockage or leaking (haemorrhage) of a blood vessel in the brain. As a result, the area of brain normally served by the blood vessel dies off and, in the case of a haemorrhage, additional brain damage is done to the tissues surrounding the leak. Large strokes are often fatal but many people survive smaller strokes that do not affect the most critical parts of the brain. As a result people can develop problems such as language difficulty (aphasia) or any of the other problems also seen in dementia. Brain damage from injury in accidents is another problem affecting significant numbers of people each year.

That the cause of the brain function abnormalities in these conditions is not dementia would probably be obvious from the history, particularly the suddenness with which stroke or injury occurs. It is not always so straightforward, however, to distinguish dementia from other conditions that can look like it. Vascular dementia can also start suddenly, following a stroke. An overview of the medical assessment of someone newly presenting with possible dementia is detailed in chapter 5.

Formal systems of disease description

In order to classify diseases and ensure as much as possible that doctors in different parts of the world are talking about the same condition there are formal systems that describe the various features of illnesses. Two main schemes exist and it is not important to know the details, but for the sake of accuracy they are called the Diagnostic and Statistic Manual, currently in version 4 (DSM-IV), which is an American-based system for classifying psychiatric conditions and the International Classification of Disease, version 10 (ICD-10), which is produced by the World Health Organisation and covers all medical conditions. Dementia is described formally in both systems and in similar ways. The description of Alzheimer's disease just listed is from the DSM-IV criteria. ICD-10 includes personality change within its description, whereas DSM-IV criteria include a 'social impact' factor, i.e. that the symptoms represent a change from a person's previous level of functioning, and that they cause a significant degree of trouble in social or even occupational circumstances.

This chapter has given a basic description of dementia. In order to understand something about why we think dementia occurs, and how it is that presently available treatments appear to work, it is useful to have some knowledge of the structure and function of the brain.

Chapter 2

The brain, ageing and dementia

Brain facts

The adult human brain weighs, on average, about 1.3 kg, or about 2 per cent of an adult's total body weight. The brain, however, consumes 16 per cent of the total energy used by the body – an amount eight times greater than expected on a weight for weight basis. The brain demands a constant supply of oxygen from the bloodstream – significant interruption of blood flow to the brain causes unconsciousness within a few seconds and at normal body temperature brain cells cannot survive more than about three minutes without oxygen. Brain cells use glucose (sugar) almost exclusively for their fuel supply, unlike most other tissues of the body that can also use fats for energy. At any one point in time brain cells store only about two minutes' worth of glucose, so they need constantly to top this up from the bloodstream.

Confusion and dementia

The brain is therefore intensely active but it is also vulnerable to many sorts of interruption. Conditions such as lack of oxygen, excess alcohol or drugs, head injury and severe infection among many others can cause sudden-onset confusion or *delirium*. If the cause of the change in brain function in someone who is delirious is found and dealt with then the delirium may disappear completely.

Unfortunately the same is not true in dementia and even our best available treatments have only a small impact on the muddled thinking that can accompany the condition. People with dementia are more prone to delirium than people whose brain is normal. When a person with dementia's function changes rapidly, delirium caused by a correctable factor may be to blame. Depression, for example, commonly accompanies dementia and effective treatment of it can significantly improve someone's ability to cope with life.

Most people with dementia are elderly, who as a group tend to have multiple medical problems. This can lead to increasing numbers of drugs being prescribed with secondary problems arising from interactions between the drugs or mistakes being made in taking them. Excess alcohol intake or the development of another medical condition that is masked by the symptoms of dementia are other ways in which someone with dementia may become worse. It is easy to blame dementia for every aspect of someone's behaviour and one needs to be alert to the possibility of some other explanation, especially if there is a change over a short period of time.

Brain structure

Figure 1 shows the general structure of the brain. The right and left halves (hemispheres) are extensively interconnected by nerve fibres that relay messages to and from different parts of the brain and, via the spinal cord, every part of the body. The surface layer of each hemisphere of the brain, the so-called 'grey matter' is folded and made up mainly of nerve cells, called neurones. There are over

Figure 1: Brain structure – nerve cells (neurones) within the brain are connected in multiple ways with each other and, through the spinal cord, with others parts of the body

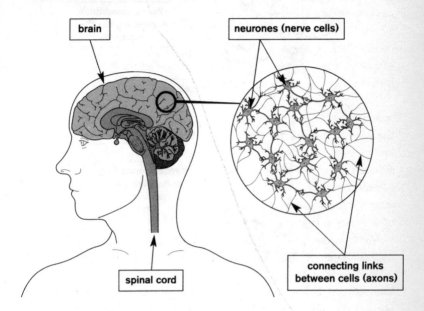

100 billion neurones in the brain and nervous system of a human being, each only a few thousandths of a millimetre across. An individual neurone is shown in diagrammatic form in figure 2. From the cell body a single main nerve fibre arises, which conducts the signals arising from this particular neurone. This fibre divides into many smaller branches, which in turn eventually make contact with other neurones. Each neurone also receives signals from other neurones through fibres connected to its cell body. The network of connections between nerve cells is enormously complex – there are said to be more possible ways for the neurones in one person to link up than there are atoms in the Universe. Signals travelling between nerve cells are all that let us think, see, hear, imagine, feel, memorise, recall, feel emotion and everything else. We have barely begun to understand this incredible process.

Figure 2: The structure of a neurone

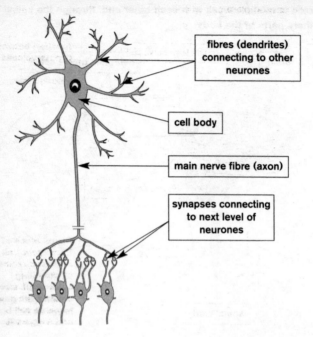

fibres (dendrites) connecting to other neurones

cell body

main nerve fibre (axon)

synapses connecting to next level of neurones

Nerve signalling

Although brain cells and nerves are a bit like electrical cables and switches in the way they pass signals around, they in fact use a combination of electrical impulses and chemical reactions to deliver their messages to each other. Where a fibre from one neurone reaches another the fibre ending spreads out to form a highly specialised connection zone – the 'synapse'. Here the fibre and the next cell are very close to each other, but they do not actually touch. This is illustrated in figure 3.

Within the nerve fibre ending there are microscopic 'packets' of a particular chemical compound held in readiness. When the first neurone sends a signal for whatever reason and this reaches the

Figure 3: Junction between nerve cells (synapse) showing the way signals are passed from cell to cell

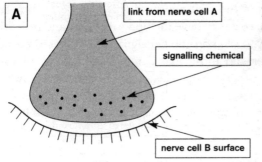

Junction between two nerve cells (synapse) – resting state.

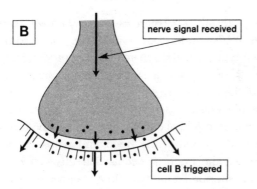

Signal received from nerve cell A causes release of signalling compound, which crosses the gap to nerve cell B and triggers it.

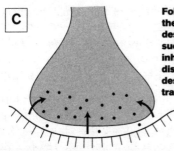

Following the signal, free chemical in the gap is taken back by cell A or destroyed by the activity of enzymes such as cholinesterase. Cholinesterase inhibitor drugs used in Alzheimer's disease slow down this enzyme destruction, thus improving the transmission of nerve signals.

synapse at the end of its connecting fibre tiny amounts of this signalling chemical are released into the gap between it and the surface of the next nerve cell. The chemical crosses the gap and triggers a reaction in the next neurone. This may be to stimulate the next cell to fire or it may have the opposite effect and make the next cell less likely to send on another signal. The balance between signals that trigger and those that dampen the activity of each neurone changes continuously. This is the complicated way that nerve cells communicate with each other. The chemicals used by the nervous system to carry out this signalling process are known as neurotransmitters.

Neurotransmitters

Many individual neurotransmitter substances are now known, and the actions they have are also understood to a degree. Within some parts of the brain one type of neurotransmitter may predominate over others, whereas in other areas a range of neurotransmitters may all be used by different neurones.

In the context of dementia it is helpful to know about one particular neurotransmitter, called acetyl choline. Acetyl choline is manufactured by cells deep within the brain and whose nerve fibres extend throughout the brain. It seems that this system is particularly important in supporting memory. In Alzheimer's disease the number of these acetyl choline producing brain cells is much reduced. One of the ways in which Alzheimer's disease is now treated is with drugs to boost the effect of the remaining acetyl choline producing cells in the brain.

Computers and brains

In a crude way computers mimic brain function. They have input devices such as keyboards whereas we have our senses. Computers have memory storage, as do we (although it's less clear how ours works), and programs of instruction which are like our learning and experience, which tell us how to get things done. The powerhouse of a computer is the central chip that can do billions of calculations a second. The biological equivalent is the continuous chatter of signals between neurones that somehow achieves something like the same end.

The calculating power of computers can be increased by connecting many of them together and getting them to work simultaneously on the same problem. The brain appears also to use this principle of 'parallel processing' in a way, so that various parts of the brain may at any time be contributing to carrying out a particular task. If a part of the brain is damaged then sometimes other areas can be recruited to make up some of the deficit, which is why many people with significant brain injury can make a remarkable recovery. Although in people with dementia some parts of the brain may be more affected than others, it is basically a diffuse brain disease and, while people can fluctuate to some extent, spontaneous improvement does not occur.

Adaptability of nerve connections

Within a computer the various components and wires are all permanently fixed to each other. The 'wiring' in a human brain is different in this important respect, because the pattern of connections between synapses is able to adapt and change. When the same action is repeated a sort of electrical pathway is laid down in the brain so that the action becomes increasingly easy. Similarly a particular memory can be thought of as a unique set of signals between a specific group of brain cells. If this memory relates to an experience that is often repeated then the connections become stronger and the memory is reinforced.

This ability of nerve cell connections to change with time and in response to experience is called 'synaptic plasticity' and it is what makes it possible for an experience to turn into a memory that can later be recalled. Loss of synaptic plasticity is a key feature of dementia. An analogy is the thread that shows the way out of the labyrinth. In dementia a person is unable to lay this thread, and their memories get lost.

This simple explanation of brain function misses out a lot that we know, and even more that we are still to learn, but it serves as the background against which we can try to understand what goes on in dementia.

Normal ageing

Brain cells are not replaced when they wear out and die, as they do naturally from early adulthood onwards. In elderly people some loss of brain cells is therefore normal. Loss of water and supporting tissue also contributes to the normal degree of shrinkage seen in the healthy older brain. Looking at the fine details of brain structure in normal ageing one sees also that there is a drop in the number of connections (synapses) each cell makes with its neighbours. Nerve cells become slower to respond to signals and to pass on signals down the line. All of these effects combine to make it normal for an older person to have slower response times and some memory loss.

Two additional changes are also seen in the brain in normal ageing:

1 The accumulation of protein material that arises from the death of other brain cells. These protein collections are called 'plaques' (or 'senile plaques' although their presence does not necessarily imply senility!).
2 Small spiral-shaped proteins called neurofibrillary tangles, or 'NFTs'. These develop in damaged neurones. In normal, healthy neurones the cell structures NFTs arise from are involved in making neurotransmitters available at the nerve synapses.

Small amounts of senile plaques and to a lesser extent of NFTs are seen in samples of brain tissue from people with no evidence of dementia.

Changes seen in dementia

In all people with dementia there is a much greater loss of neurones than normal. There are also features that distinguish the different types of dementia from each other and which can be seen when examining brain tissue in detail. In the remaining part of this chapter brief descriptions are given of these features, as they are helpful in understanding dementia. However, we've already made the point that dementia is diagnosed clinically, i.e. by its effects on a person's memory and functioning. Dementia is *not* diagnosed by specialists looking down microscopes at samples of brain. In the next chapter we therefore start to look at dementia from a more practical viewpoint, through its impact on daily life and what one can do about it.

ALZHEIMER'S DISEASE

Alzheimer's disease is the underlying cause in about 60 per cent of all people with dementia in the UK. In Alzheimer's disease the typical changes within the brain include many more senile plaques and, especially, neurofibrillary tangles than are seen in normal ageing. The distribution of the loss of neurones is also different, with some parts of the brain more affected than others. Regions deep within each hemisphere of the brain, called the hippocampi, show particular loss of neurones and these regions are known from other brain studies to be important to memory function. The nerves connecting the hippocampi to the rest of the brain predominantly use acetyl choline as their neurotransmitter.

VASCULAR DEMENTIA

Five per cent of people with dementia have a type that is accounted for by brain damage due to poor circulation of blood to the brain, or more correctly the results of a large stroke or multiple small strokes causing loss of brain tissue. This is known as Vascular

Dementia (see chapter 3 for more on vascular disease). It is commoner to have a combination of features of both Alzheimer's disease and vascular dementia together, rather than vascular dementia alone. About 15 per cent of people with dementia have this combination of causes.

DEMENTIA WITH LEWY BODIES

This type of dementia gets its name from the appearance of some neurones when examined under the microscope. These cells were first described in a different region of the brain responsible for Parkinson's disease, by a German-American neurologist called Friedrich Lewy in 1914. 'Lewy bodies' are small particles seen within affected neurones. (Lewy's contemporaries were also famous names in the history of brain disease. He worked in Alois Alzheimer's laboratory in Munich, beside Hans Creutzfeldt and Alfons Jakob. Creutzfeldt-Jakob disease, or CJD, is a rare cause of dementia caused by 'prion' protein from infected tissue.)

Parkinson's disease, for which the old term was 'shaking palsy', is a disorder affecting muscle control that causes tremor, muscle stiffness and slowness of movement. Although it is not a form of dementia there is some overlap between the symptoms of it and Lewy body dementia. Lewy body disease is estimated to account for about 10 per cent of people with dementia.

OTHER CAUSES

Between them Alzheimer's disease, vascular dementia and dementia with Lewy bodies account for 90 per cent of affected people. Of the remaining 10 per cent there is a considerable number of causes. The priority when someone initially appears to show signs of dementia is to search for other possible explanations for their symptoms. In up to 5 per cent of people another medical illness will be found responsible. The range of possible medical causes of dementia-like symptoms is very wide but some of the main ones include severe under-activity of the thyroid gland, brain tumours or raised pressure of the fluid that surrounds the brain, some types of vitamin deficiency, and alcoholism. Some of these causes are treatable but only about one person in 50 with apparent dementia will be found to have a correctable cause for it.

The final 5 per cent of people with dementia have one of the rare causes such as fronto-temporal degeneration or Pick's disease. In the earlier stages of Pick's disease memory is less affected than in Alzheimer's disease but instead there may be more marked personality changes. As time goes by it becomes more like Alzheimer's disease.

Establishing the type of dementia

Making an accurate diagnosis of the type of dementia is important, especially when someone is being assessed for the first time. Occasionally a correctable condition is revealed. More commonly it is not, but the treatments we have available for dementia do not work across the board. Dementia with Lewy bodies and Pick's disease do not respond to treatments that help Alzheimer's disease, for example. Pure vascular dementia may be helped by different treatment to Alzheimer's disease but if the conditions co-exist in one person then both need to be covered.

As we will see, a truly accurate diagnosis of dementia is more of an aim than an achievable goal in most people. The tools we have for diagnosis are relatively crude and in practice treatments are sometimes given simply because we can't always be sure that they will or will not do any good.

Chapter 3

The causes of dementia

Alzheimer's disease

In the last chapter mention was made that in Alzheimer's disease an accumulation occurs of material in the brain. This takes two forms: plaques and neurofibrillary tangles. It's worth noting a bit more detail about these substances. Plaques are comprised of the remnants of old neurones mixed with a protein substance called amyloid. Neurofibrillary tangles are also made of protein, this time in the form of tightly wound spiral strands. The protein that NFTs are made from is called tau (rhymes with *how*). Plaques and NFTs are seen in small amounts in normal brain tissue but they are much more abundant in Alzheimer's disease. This is particularly true of NFTs. It seems likely that excess amounts of these proteins impair the ability of nerve fibres to signal to each other, so understanding what causes them to build up would help explain Alzheimer's disease.

GENES

A small number of people develop dementia of Alzheimer's type at an earlier age than usual, before 65, and a proportion of them pass the tendency for dementia on to their offspring. Gene tests have revealed several 'faulty' genes that are associated with the occurrence of early-onset Alzheimer's disease, such as the gene that controls the manufacture within the body of the protein a stage before amyloid (amyloid precursor protein, or APP) and two others called 'presenilins' - PS1 and PS2.

When one looks at the older population of people, who make up by far the majority of people with Alzheimer's disease, less is known of any gene faults that increase risk. One that seems important concerns the gene that determines the production in the body of a protein involved in transporting cholesterol around in the blood, called apolipoprotein E (APOE). The presence of some types of APOE may speed up the onset of Alzheimer's disease, but do not cause it. There is, however, other support for a genetic link to the cause of older-onset Alzheimer disease, through family histories. The first-degree relative (sibling or child) of someone with Alzheimer's disease has an increased chance of developing the disease. However, this does not mean he or she will necessarily do so, because the risk only becomes apparent if they live long enough (age 90 or beyond) and do not die as a result of something else first. Unless someone has a large number of very elderly close relatives then even someone with a strong family tendency towards developing Alzheimer's disease would not be aware of the fact. Most people with Alzheimer's disease therefore do not have such a family history.

In the majority of medical conditions in which heredity plays a part it is not possible to predict with certainty who will and will not get the condition. Instead, what people inherit through their genes is a *potential* tendency to develop the condition, and whether they then do so depends on whether they are exposed to some extra, triggering, factors in the course of their life. This seems to be true of asthma, diabetes, high blood pressure, arthritis and many other conditions, including Alzheimer's disease. What the trigger factors are for dementia (and indeed for the other diseases) is largely speculation. It could be infection from viruses or exposure to certain chemicals or even stress in the case of some conditions. The part genes play is to set up the background level of risk. It is therefore possible that someone at a genetically high risk of developing Alzheimer's disease never does so because they never come into contact with one of the trigger factors.

Genetic changes are therefore thought to be significantly involved among the causes of Alzheimer's disease but exactly how and why are still largely matters of research. More detail than this is probably not of great interest to the general reader and it is important to emphasise that genetic testing is of no use in telling the ordinary individual how likely they are to develop Alzheimer's disease. The exceptions are those families in which there are several members whose dementia appeared at a very young age (40s or 50s); people from such families should be advised by an expert in genetic disease.

OTHER CAUSES

There are other theories concerning the cause of Alzheimer's disease, which probably tie up with the gene theories although we presently do not know enough about either to know how. One concerns the fact that the tau proteins in neurofibrillary tangles are chemically changed so that they are more tightly bound to each other. This makes them less efficient in delivering neurotransmitter molecules to where they are needed within the neurones. It also may be the case that when individual neurones die, as they do naturally, they may leave behind remnant compounds that are toxic to the surrounding healthy cells. The mechanism that normally mops up such compounds, known as free radicals, may be faulty in Alzheimer's disease, so healthy neurones effectively become poisoned.

RISK FACTORS FOR ALZHEIMER'S DISEASE

A 'risk factor' for a condition is a situation or event that, if present, raises the chance that the other condition will occur. Skiing is a risk factor for breaking a leg and bereavement is a risk factor for depression. In Alzheimer's disease the strongest risk factor is being elderly. Alzheimer's disease is also more common in elderly women than in elderly men, even after one accounts for the fact that more women than men live to an advanced age. A family history of Alzheimer's disease, as just mentioned, is another risk factor. None of these links explains the cause of the condition – risk factors are just observed relationships and sometimes the reasons for the links are not clear.

Vascular disease

The second commonest type of dementia seen in the UK is that secondary to the brain damage that arises from strokes. A stroke occurs when the blood supply to an area of brain is closed, either by a clot within the artery supplying blood to that region of the brain or as a result of leakage from a burst artery. The area of brain served by that blood vessel therefore dies. We'll come back in more detail shortly to the relevance this has to dementia but first we should go over the background to why it is that blood vessels may block or burst open, as this makes it easier to understand the rationale behind one of the main aspects of dementia treatment, which aims to reduce the likelihood of more strokes occurring.

ARTERIES AND VEINS

'Vascular' is the medical word that means 'to do with the blood vessels'. There are two types of blood vessel – *arteries* that take blood rich in oxygen and under high pressure from the heart and deliver it to every part of the body and *veins* that return the blood back to the lungs and heart to be charged up with oxygen again. Apart from the fact that veins can bulge (become 'varicose') there

Figure 4: Healthy and diseased arteries

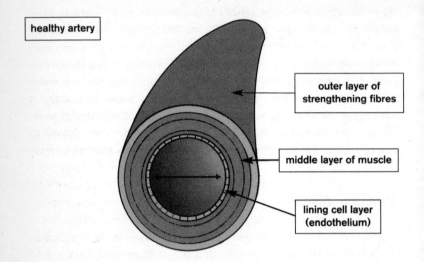

healthy artery

outer layer of strengthening fibres

middle layer of muscle

lining cell layer (endothelium)

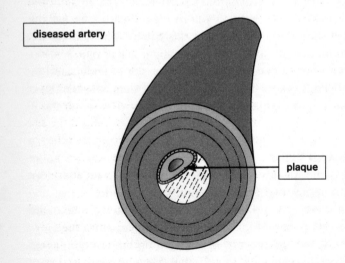

diseased artery

plaque

are few diseases of the veins of any importance. Arteries are, however, a completely different story. Arteries are prone to furring up as we get older, a process that we commonly call 'hardening of the arteries' and which is properly termed 'atherosclerosis'.

Atherosclerosis

If you took two arteries, one healthy and one affected by atherosclerosis, cut them across and then inspected each under a microscope you would see something like that shown in figure 4. The normal artery is above, with a wide channel for the blood to flow through. Arteries are tubes of muscle with a special interior lining of cells that ensures blood normally flows along very smoothly. Below is the diseased artery, substantially narrowed by thickening of the muscle layer and in particular by a fatty deposit that has built up under the lining. (This is also called plaque but it is quite a different substance from the plaque that we mentioned in connection with Alzheimer's disease. Nor does it have anything to do with unbrushed teeth!)

Plaque in arteries is a mixture of fats, particularly cholesterol, as well as a build-up of cells from the body's immune system and proteins like those that form in a scar. A plaque starts off small but with time it gets bigger, steadily narrowing the artery at this point. As well as causing an obstruction to blood flow, a plaque is also a weak point in an artery. In particular the thin covering of the plaque can rupture, exposing it and the underlying muscular layer of the artery. This can trigger another sequence of chemical reactions in the blood, which results in the blood clotting at the site of the plaque rupture. This is very often what occurs in a stroke (or a heart attack if it occurs inside one of the heart's arteries rather than in the brain). Suddenly what had been a narrowed artery can rapidly turn into a completely blocked one.

Because the pressure of the blood within an artery is high and because the artery is weak at these points then the artery may give way, allowing blood to escape into the surrounding brain tissue. Not only does this mean that blood is not going forwards to deliver oxygen to the brain area normally served by the artery but there is extra brain damage from the high-pressure blood leaking out. This is called a brain haemorrhage, and it can be extremely dangerous. Of the two types of stroke, those due to blockage of an artery in the brain are commoner than those due to haemorrhage but the underlying cause of both is usually atherosclerosis. Some people may have weak points in the arteries that are not due to athero-sclerosis but instead may have been present all their lives. For one reason or another these might rupture in adulthood and cause similar effects.

The other important cause of artery blockage occurs when small clots arising from some other part of the blood vessel system end up in a brain artery and jam there, blocking it. Such clots, which may be of very small size, can arise in certain situations more commonly than others. The most important is when the major arteries within the neck that supply blood to the brain are them-selves furred up extensively with plaque that sends showers of tiny clots from its surface.

When a clot travels from one part of the blood vessel system to another it is called an 'embolism' and the other major cause of embolism causing strokes is a condition of irregular beating of the heart called atrial fibrillation. In this condition, which is fairly common in older people, the normal co-ordination of the beating of the heart's chambers is lost. The heart still beats away but it does so irregularly instead of with a steady rhythm. As a result, tiny eddy currents of blood occur within the chambers of the heart. In these regions small blood clots can form which are then swept out into the general circulation. They then may get stuck within a critical part of the body's network of arteries, such as in the brain. Sometimes one of these clots will stick only for a short time – perhaps a few hours – during which time the person may experi-ence symptoms as serious as paralysis. Then the clot breaks up or is dissolved by the body's own defences against such events and the symptoms clear. These are called 'transient ischaemic attacks', the word 'ischaemia' being the medical term for 'lack of blood supply'. Someone who experiences a 'TIA', as they are commonly known, is at high risk of going on to have a permanent stroke within a few weeks or months.

Risk factors for atherosclerosis and vascular dementia
Some degree of atherosclerosis is probably an inevitable part of ageing but there are many recognised risk factors associated with premature or more severe artery hardening. These are also risk factors for developing vascular dementia. Chief among these are:

- high blood pressure
- a high level of cholesterol in the blood
- smoking
- diabetes

We'll return to these issues in chapter 6 when we look in more detail at dementia treatments.

Strokes and dementia

There are some parts of the brain in which even a small stroke can be fatal, for example in the region at the top of the spinal cord in which there are the vital areas controlling breathing (called the brain stem). If, however, a stroke occurs higher up in the wiring, so to speak, of the brain then even quite a large amount of brain damage may still be compatible with the person surviving. The results of the stroke will, however, depend very much on the area of brain affected. One common scenario is loss of power down part or all of one side of the body. Such a split occurs because the nerve fibres of the right and left halves of the brain which go to the spinal cord swap sides along the way. The right half of the brain therefore controls the left half of the body, and vice versa. It is quite possible for someone to have a stroke of this nature and retain normal higher mental function or perhaps have only one or two specific difficulties such as difficulty expressing themselves in speech. Others, who as a result of a stroke have more substantial brain damage in key areas, may have all the symptoms of dementia.

THE EFFECT OF MULTIPLE SMALL STROKES

The dramatic sort of stroke described above is a good enough example to use when describing the basic process that goes on, and most people are familiar with the fact that strokes can cause such major and sudden-onset disability. However, individual strokes can also be more subtle and smaller scale.

Instead of involving the large arteries that distribute blood to wide areas of brain the smaller arteries, serving correspondingly smaller areas of brain, may also be affected by atherosclerosis. Multiple small strokes of these small arteries might never be sufficient to cause paralysis or any of the more obvious physical symptoms, but instead over a period of time they gradually reduce the amount of fully functioning brain.

An area of tissue that has been starved of its blood supply is called an 'infarct', and dementia resulting from this process of artery blockage is therefore called *multi-infarct dementia*. The other term doctors use to describe this type of dementia is *vascular dementia*.

Causes of other types of dementia

Alzheimer's disease and vascular dementia, alone or in combination with each other, account for 80 per cent of everyone affected. The third main variety of dementia is the Lewy body type, which, as mentioned earlier, has some features in common with Parkinson's disease. One of the very important findings in both Lewy body dementia and Parkinson's disease is the reduction in numbers of a specialised type of brain cell that uses a neurotransmitter called dopamine. Although Parkinson-like conditions can be caused by the side effects of some prescription drugs, poisoning from carbon monoxide or a drug of abuse called MPTP, and rarely from a type of brain infection (encephalitis), the causes of 'true' Parkinson's disease and Lewy body dementia are unknown.

As with vascular dementia and Alzheimer's disease, Lewy body dementia may co-exist with other types. Post mortem studies have shown that as many as 40 per cent of people who in life were diagnosed with Alzheimer's disease also have Lewy bodies in brain tissue samples.

The cause of Pick's disease, one of the rarer types of dementia, is unknown. Korsakoff's syndrome is a dementia-like illness caused by a deficiency of the vitamin thiamin (vitamin B1). Although such a deficiency can be caused by prolonged malnutrition this rare syndrome is usually associated with prolonged alcohol misuse as well. Giving supplements of thiamin can improve the dementia, which reinforces the need to be sure of the diagnosis.

Protection against dementia

No one knows their future, or their risk of getting any disease. Instead, we work on the principle of trying to keep healthy, taking exercise and a decent diet, not smoking, avoiding being overweight or taking too much alcohol, and so on. Doing so, we know, reduces everyone's risk of developing a range of illnesses such as diabetes, heart disease, some types of cancer and high blood pressure no matter what our genetic tendency is to any of these. Much interest has therefore been focused on identifying actions that could reduce the risk of anyone getting dementia. The results have been mixed and in some cases rather confusing.

NON-STEROIDAL ANTI-INFLAMMATORY DRUGS

In many conditions such as arthritis the affected tissues, in this case the joints, are inflamed. Drugs capable of reducing this inflammation therefore act to soothe the pain, heat and swelling that accompany the arthritis. Steroid drugs are the most powerful anti-inflammatories but their use for longer than a few weeks is often accompanied by many undesirable side effects. The first non-steroidal anti-inflammatory drug (NSAID) was aspirin but this too has potential side effects that limit its routine use as a painkiller. Ibuprofen and drugs like it are the modern 'NSAIDs' and are among the most commonly used of all drugs. Early studies suggested that people taking NSAIDs regularly were at less risk of developing Alzheimer's disease than those who did not, but more recent studies have not confirmed this. NSAIDs are of no benefit in reducing the symptoms of Alzheimer's disease in those who already have the condition. Research into the possibility that some of the newer types of NSAIDs might slow the progress of dementia is in progress but it will be years before the results are known.

HORMONE REPLACEMENT THERAPY

The use of supplements of the 'female hormones' oestrogen, with or without progesterone, to alleviate the symptoms of the menopause in women is more familiarly known as HRT. Until recently (2002), one of the benefits of HRT was thought to be a degree of protection from Alzheimer's disease. More recent evidence has not only failed to confirm this but has suggested the opposite effect – that it may increase the risk when started at the menopause. The evidence that HRT is beneficial in general terms to women who have an early menopause (younger than 45) remains convincing but its use in post-menopausal women has been clouded in doubt since the publication of the results of several large research trials in 2002. It can no longer be considered any protection against the onset of dementia.

Whether men suffer from a 'male menopause' is a controversial issue that is beyond the scope of this book. Some men do appear to suffer symptoms in middle age or older that are alleviated by the male equivalent of HRT, which is testosterone replacement. A small amount of evidence suggests that some of these men benefit in terms of mental function too, but there is no evidence to suggest any protection against the development of dementia from such treatment.

ANTIOXIDANTS

The body constantly reacts with oxygen as part of the energy producing process within cells. As a consequence of this activity, highly reactive molecules are produced known as free radicals. These interact with other molecules within the cell and can cause 'oxidative damage' to proteins, cell membranes and genes. This damage has been implicated in the cause of many diseases including cancers and it has an impact on the body's ageing process. The toxic effects of free radicals on brain cells may be part of the process of Alzheimer's disease.

It's the job of antioxidants to neutralise free radicals and the body produces an armoury of them to defend itself. The metabolic processes that produce antioxidants are controlled and influenced by an individual's genetic make-up and the extra environmental factors (such as diet, smoking and pollution) to which your body is exposed. Unfortunately, changes in our lifestyles which include more environmental pollution and less quality in our diets, mean that we are exposed to more free radicals than ever before. Our internal production of antioxidants is insufficient to neutralise and scavenge all the free radicals but there is an abundant supply of antioxidants in a wide variety of foods. By increasing our dietary intake of antioxidants, we can help our body to defend itself.

Examples of food-based antioxidants include vitamins (vitamin E, vitamin C, and beta carotene) and the trace elements that are components of antioxidant enzymes (including selenium, copper, zinc and manganese) amongst others. A diet rich in fruit and vegetables will normally supply all the extra antioxidants that we need.

Studies using vitamin E have again not shown a protective effect as such but have suggested an ability of this vitamin to slow down the rate of deterioration in people with moderate to severe Alzheimer's disease.

VACCINATION

This is still at the research stage and there have been setbacks in early trials but the principle is to develop a vaccine against the amyloid protein that builds up in Alzheimer's disease (and to some extent also in vascular and Lewy body dementias). Vaccination is based on the principle of making the body's immune system sensitive to foreign material – usually bacteria or viruses as most vaccines are for protection against infectious disease. However, if the amyloid protein were recognised as foreign by the immune system and cleared away before it built up then we might have an effective form of protection suitable for widespread use.

REDUCING THE RISKS FOR VASCULAR DEMENTIA

If someone with high blood pressure has this well controlled then their subsequent risk of major stroke is considerably reduced. Similarly, lowering high levels of blood cholesterol and stopping smoking reduce the progress of atherosclerosis and these have well-documented benefits in preventing related diseases such as heart attacks.

As atherosclerosis can lead to vascular dementia good control of all these 'cardiovascular risk factors' should reduce the likelihood that vascular dementia will occur. Despite the good sense this makes it has been hard to prove. Partly this is because people at high risk of developing cardiovascular diseases are likely to die from them before they reach an age at which dementia will appear. It is also because dementia purely due to vascular disease is not as common as dementia due to the combination of vascular disease and Alzheimer's disease and the latter is unaffected by efforts to improve the former. Nonetheless there is enough evidence to state that the lowering of high blood cholesterol and reduction of other risks such as high blood pressure are worthwhile in slowing the pace of vascular or mixed dementia. As we'll come to in the next chapter, it is difficult or impossible to neatly separate out the different possible causes of dementia in real life, so this means that any person with dementia who also has significant cardiovascular risk factors should be treated for those risk factors unless, for other reasons, to do so would be impractical or inappropriate. In the case of people over 80 we do not presently have enough information to say whether treatment with statins, and other cardiovascular risk-reducing treatments, are definitely valuable.

More research needed!

In all honesty the preceding section has not been particularly enlightening. About the only safe statement that can be made about what can be done to guard against dementia is that we don't know for sure. Some ways that seemed promising, like the use of HRT, now look like damp squibs. Others, like antioxidant vitamins, might be worthwhile but we haven't enough evidence. Vaccines are still a long way off and might not succeed anyway. This is pretty much the same picture as in many other important medical conditions. Dementia has not been the most attractive subject for research funding for most of the past few decades. It is now on the map because the numbers of people with the condition are increasing to levels that cannot be ignored and because the costs of providing care for dementia sufferers are high. The pharmaceutical industry has also become interested in putting money into drug research for dementia.

This is all to the good as far as the profile of dementia is concerned, but research will still be difficult even if more cash is available. If the increasing number of people with dementia is due to a complex interaction between environmental factors and genetics, it is very difficult to work out the most important components of that combination. We really have no idea what might be the most important risk factors in the environment, and as we saw earlier our understanding of the genetics of dementia is still basic. If diet is important, as seems likely, we need to know also if it matters when in life this is so. It could, for example, be that what we eat in our teenage years matters more than what we eat as adults. If vitamin supplements are helpful then at what age should one start taking them? What is the best dose, and for how long should they be taken? We do not have any of these answers. Conducting research into the possible causes of dementia requires large studies extending over long time scales and involving large numbers of people from different backgrounds. It is very difficult indeed.

Taking the global view

Clearly our present knowledge of how to prevent dementia is very inadequate. The same can be said for most if not all other major medical conditions though and this does not mean we have no idea of what to do.

The first approach is to take a more global view of our health rather than trying to come up with a specific strategy for dementia, another for diabetes, and another for cancer, etc. There is plenty of evidence to suggest that most of the actions that can help protect against dementia are the same as those that help promote healthy living in general. A good regular intake of fruit and vegetables ensures enough natural antioxidants for most people. That helps protect against many types of cancer as well as dementia. Exercise improves physical and mental fitness and reduces the chance of bowel cancer and diabetes. Cutting out smoking cuts the risk of many cancers as well as reducing the occurrence of atherosclerosis. There are common themes among all these health tips, and 90 per cent of what we can do to help ourselves not get disease A is the same as for diseases B to Z.

There is no drug or treatment that presently can be said to protect against dementia. The best approach is to keep as fit in general terms as possible.

Chapter 4

Dementia diagnosis: (1) Symptoms and other considerations

The preceding chapters have set out the basic scientific information on dementia. You know by now that there are different types of dementia, although these can only be determined accurately by detailed analysis of the brain. But you will also recall that the condition is diagnosed by listening to and observing real people and not by looking down microscopes. There is no characteristic combination of symptoms that can only be Alzheimer's disease, or Lewy body dementia or vascular dementia; the symptoms all overlap. In the following sections therefore 'dementia' is used in a general sense but when certain patterns of symptoms are more suggestive of particular types of dementia this is pointed out.

Memory loss

The main problems that arise in dementia are the failure of memory recall and recognition. Memory loss is the commonest first symptom of dementia although the practicalities of how that happens are as varied as people themselves. Here are some common examples:

- She keeps repeating the same question, despite being given a clear answer.
- She has difficulty putting names to faces, eventually including those of well-known family and friends.
- She gets lost on the way to the shops, or to other familiar destinations.
- She often misplaces items such as keys, glasses, wallet.
- She forgets to pay bills, return phone calls, keep appointments.

Although distant memory is also impaired in dementia it is recent memory that goes first and to the greater degree. You might have a normal conversation with your partner about a holiday you had ten years ago and yet he might not recall accompanying you to the travel agent that morning to book your next trip, or what you both had in the café for lunch on the way back.

Language problems

Recall of experiences or facts and recognition of items or faces are memory functions. In chapter 1 the more specifically named brain function abnormalities were also mentioned. For example aphasia, the disturbance of language and word use, might appear thus:

- He hesitates as if having difficulty finding the right word to say. (Here the problem is not just of poor memory in remembering the right word but in associating the right word with the idea that he wants to put across.)
- He uses the wrong word, for example calling a cat a door.

(Difficulties are most pronounced when trying to find the right nouns and names.)
- Sentences are left incomplete or he gets lost over what he wanted to say.

Difficulties with the tasks of daily living

The combination of problems in memory, 'executive function' and in carrying out 'motor' tasks becomes most obvious in the ordinary tasks of daily living. Light switches can't be located nor is the light switched on when needed. The telephone becomes hard to use and numbers get mis-dialled. The cooker becomes an area of concern if rings or gas taps are left on or pots and kettles are boiled dry. Car driving may become an area of even greater worry as judgement becomes impaired. Money difficulties can take all sorts of forms, from lost wallets to unpaid bills or credit card misuse.

As time goes by the more basic daily tasks such as eating, drinking and self-care may become more difficult.

A rapid run through of such symptoms can give an overly pessimistic view of dementia. Although in many people all these symptoms and more may appear, most people with dementia have patchy areas of difficulty mixed with preservation of adequate or even quite normal function. One of the many aims of good dementia care is to avoid preconceived ideas about how the condition will behave in an individual. The impact of difficulties needs to be minimised, and preserved abilities and strengths need to be encouraged. The concept of 'person-centred care' is one we will return to.

Behaviour changes

Changes in a person's behaviour are very often part of the picture of dementia. Some behaviours result directly from the loss of memory, such as a tendency to wander or get lost. Others are the result of the global effect of dementia on brain function, such as repetitive speech, sleep disturbance, the neglect of eating and drinking properly. More severe brain function disturbance causes some patients to experience hallucinations – sights or sounds, or both, that are real to the person experiencing them but not happening in reality. Such hallucinations may cause the person affected to respond to them. Some types of behaviour may put the patient at increased risk, such as neglected heating in winter or financial difficulties from inappropriate spending.

COPING BEHAVIOUR

In early dementia it is common for people to be aware that they are beginning to have difficulties. Both consciously and unconsciously they try to compensate for these in various ways. Problems remembering things may prompt the use of lists for example. The proper use of coping strategies can help reduce the impact of dementia.

Embarrassment over forgetfulness or getting into problems with bills may, however, mean that they conceal what is going on. In turn they might then become defensive or upset if challenged by the family about whether they are having any problems. Attempts to go over the head of someone with dementia and make arrangements on their behalf without their knowledge or co-operation may backfire, or simply get nowhere.

CHALLENGING BEHAVIOUR

Someone with dementia may be very resistant to believing this is what is wrong with them, or simply be incapable of understanding it. This may develop into paranoia as progressive attempts to help are interpreted by the patient as persecution. This can lead to all sorts of difficulties, from falling out with the neighbours to repeated inappropriate call outs of the police. Patients can become very frightened by their ideas. Medication can sometimes help to reduce the more extreme examples of such behaviour disturbance but will not remove it. Trying to make adequate care arrangements for someone with dementia who lacks insight into their condition but who is not so ill that they need compulsorily to be taken into care can become a great source of strain for carers and the health and social services.

Many types of behaviour in dementia can therefore be challenging to deal with. Aggression and other forms of abuse against carers are real hazards and they may need help from professional services in coping with it. Not all carers seek such help or admit they need it. The traffic is not all one way in this important but sensitive area, and the extent of abuse of people who have dementia is unknown. Some of it is malicious but more is likely to come from strain and frustration generated by the difficulties that dementia can cause.

Practical difficulties with more severely affected people with dementia can include incontinence, agitation, 'sundowning', in which the affected person becomes more disoriented and active in the late evening or turns night into day, and a host of circumstances in which risks to the person and those around them are increased.

The treatment of behavioural disturbance in dementia is dealt with in chapter 8.

Mood

Earlier we mentioned how important it is, both at the stage of initial diagnosis and later in the course of the illness, to seek and find other causes of dementia-like symptoms. Depression is the most important and commonest condition to think of in this context. It can both mimic dementia and complicate it. Successful treatment of depression in someone with dementia may substantially improve their overall functioning. Failure to recognise and treat significant depression will make other efforts to treat dementia difficult if not useless.

Anxiety is the other main type of mood disturbance that can accompany dementia, and both anxiety and depression can and very often do co-exist.

Depression in the elderly

Although depression is the commonest adult mental health problem it is often poorly detected. Apart from the stigma that attaches to mental health issues in our society, which can make people reluctant to admit they have such a problem and so seek help for it, the detection rate in elderly people is lower than for younger adults. Elderly people are less likely to volunteer that they feel depressed and both carers and health professionals are less likely to ask them. Co-existing illness, including dementia, is more common in the elderly and can itself be an important reason for depression to arise or be made worse. Bereavement (including of a pet), family separation, a past history of depression, financial difficulties, moving house, neighbour problems, social isolation and being a carer (especially for someone else with dementia) are all examples of situations that either make depression more likely to occur or which can precipitate a crisis. While temporary sadness often happens, depression is never a normal feature of old age.

SYMPTOMS OF DEPRESSION
The exact picture varies between individuals and there may be few or many of the symptoms in this list:

- low mood
- feeling of helplessness or despondency
- lack of interest in previously enjoyed activities
- anxiety
- agitation
- fatigue
- memory loss
- poor concentration
- disturbed sleep
- disturbed appetite

There are therefore many symptoms that could just as well indicate dementia, especially in its early stages when the affected person still has significant insight into what is happening to them.

Unusual presentations of depression are commoner in older people. Pre-occupation with pain or concentration on physical health problems might be the only sign of depression in old people. Emotional liability after a stroke is also common.

RECOGNISING DEPRESSION IN EARLY DEMENTIA

The first requirement is usually to think about the possibility of depression in an older person. Just asking them might be all that's needed to detect it and start the ball rolling. Talking about depression is almost always helpful and welcomed by the depressed person. Health professionals can use one of many types of question-naire to help recognise depression and although they are not essential they are helpful in suggesting the sort of questions to ask.

For example, the 'Two Question Test' is:

1 During the last month, have you often been bothered by feeling down, depressed or hopeless? (Yes/No)
2 During the last month, have you often been bothered by little interest or pleasure in doing things? (Yes/No)

A 'yes' answer to one or both of these questions makes depression likely.

The 'Geriatric Depression Scale' is:

1 Are you basically satisfied with your life? (Score 1 for No)
2 Do you feel that your life is empty? (Score 1 for Yes)
3 Are you afraid that something bad is going to happen to you? (Score 1 for Yes)
4 Do you feel happy most of the time? (Score 1 for No)

A score of 2 or more suggests depression.

RECOGNISING DEPRESSION IN LATE DEMENTIA

The above questionnaires are likely to be difficult or impossible to do in the later stages of dementia and the detection of depression in these circumstances is far from an exact science. Awareness of the possibility that depression is present is still the first requirement for making the diagnosis. The observations of many people such as carers, GP, community psychiatric nurse and voluntary helpers can all be valuable. It helps to know that depression is more likely to follow changes in routine, such as relocation (perhaps to a residential care placement), or if there has been a bereavement or other important event. Changes in drug therapy might also precipitate mood change. A change in the rate of decline in dementia can be a key feature which helps identify depression in late dementia.

At times it will not be possible to come to a firm conclusion on whether depression (or anxiety) is or is not present among all the other symptoms of dementia. In those circumstances the best option may be to give a trial of anti-depressant drug therapy. Anti-depressant drugs can have side effects that have more impact on older people than the same drugs used in younger age groups and there may also be possible interactions with other drugs to take into account (including drugs given for dementia). Apart from the technical aspects of prescribing, which can require the advice of a Consultant in Old Age Psychiatry, there can be ethical considerations too about the patient's ability to understand what is being prescribed for them and whether they can give informed consent to agree to such treatment.

When the presence of depression along with dementia is in doubt there may be good reason to consider at least a 'trial of treatment' for several weeks. During that time if there is no improvement then a decision needs to be made to either try another type of anti-depressant or discontinue the treatment.

Involving the patient

In these short books it is necessary to summarise what is often a large amount of information, with the intention of producing something that is useful both to the person with the illness and to those who know or care for them. Dementia is different to many other medical topics as it is in the nature of the illness that the patient becomes progressively less able to direct their own affairs and to make decisions for themselves on their medical care. Several times throughout the text the person with dementia is referred to as the 'patient' or in the third person. This is not intended in any way to sideline the importance of the individual with dementia.

In making a diagnosis of dementia the observations of relatives, friends and carers is invaluable, and often indispensable if the patient is not capable of giving an account on their own. Although for practical reasons it may be difficult or impossible to engage the patient fully in such decision making it should be a basic principle of dementia care that the affected person is valued and their opinion respected. Wherever possible they should be involved in their care, if they wish it.

Studies of what people with dementia want, and what their carers find helpful, repeatedly show that they value being informed about their condition and about what it means to them now and in the future. It is therefore an important part of coming to terms with dementia that there is openness about the diagnosis, discussion at an early stage about how the illness may evolve, what treatments are available, what their pros and cons are and what should be done to plan for the future. As with depression, it is far better to face up to the facts than to try to bury or dismiss them.

In the next chapter we move past the stage of initially suspecting that dementia is present to some of the more formal types of assessment used by health professionals in diagnosing the condition.

Chapter 5

Dementia diagnosis: (2) Tests

Assessing intellectual function

The most valuable part of the initial assessment of dementia is the history of the symptoms and how they have developed over the preceding months or years. From the patterns of these it may be obvious that dementia is the likely underlying cause. The observations of carers are usually helpful and are often essential to this evaluation.

Several tests, in the form mainly of questionnaires or task-based items, have been developed over the years that can be used by health professionals to assess intellectual function in a more standardised way. These are called tests of 'cognitive function'. The test in most common use for this purpose in dementia is called the 'Mini Mental State Examination' or MMSE for short.

MMSE

The MMSE is a short questionnaire with eight sections. Each contains one or more questions designed to test:

- *Orientation*
  Location questions are asked, such as 'What is today's date?' and 'What town or city are we in?'
- *Recall*
  A sequence of words is spoken, which the patient has to repeat back. The same sequence is requested of the patient after some other parts of the test have been done.
- *Attention and calculation*
  The 'serial sevens' test starts with the number 100 and then the patient has to count back by steps of 7 at a time. Then they must spell a given word backwards.
- *Language*
  Some common objects (a watch, a pen) are presented and their names requested. A phrase is stated that needs to be repeated back. Written instructions for a simple task have to be followed.
- *Motor abilities*
  A piece of paper has to be folded according to verbal instructions from the tester. A sentence needs to be written out and a drawing of intersecting pentagons needs to be copied.

The answers are accorded points, the total score possible in the MMSE being 30. The significance of the score has to be interpreted to some extent according to someone's previous mental abilities but in general a score of 24 or less is low. The MMSE score has been widely used in determining which patients are suitable for treatment with the drugs for mild to moderate dementia (see chapter 6).

Other mental function tests

Many other 'tests' like the MMSE have been developed. Despite its common use the MMSE is insensitive to picking up Alzheimer's disease at an early stage. This is because it does not contain any test of 'executive function' and it also uses very simple tasks for memory and language that fail to detect deficits until they are advanced. The Addenbrooke's Cognitive Examination (ACE) is a modification of the MMSE that expands the memory, language and visual/spatial components, and adds tests of verbal fluency. One of the significant additions that is not in the MMSE is the 'clock drawing' test. Many specialists use combinations of simple 'cognitive tests' that can be as useful as the ACE.

CLOCK DRAWING TEST

The ability to draw a clock face is sensitive to impairment of brain function as seen in dementia. Figure 5 shows a typical clock face that might be drawn by someone with dementia. In this example they have been also asked to draw the hands to show the time at ten past five. The lower value numbers are too spaced out, crowding the higher numbers and the time is wrongly shown.

Use of tests of mental function

The conditions under which these 'cognitive tests' are conducted, as well as the experience of the tester in carrying them out, are important parts of their reliability. The MMSE and tests like it are increasingly being used by GPs, nurses and other members of the primary care team because they are helpful in picking up patients who might need more investigation for suspected dementia. They are easy and quick to do and are suitable for use by professionals who are not formally trained in psychological testing. Although a GP can make a preliminary assessment of someone newly presenting with dementia and will very often be accurate in making

Figure 5: A typical clock drawing test done by someone with dementia

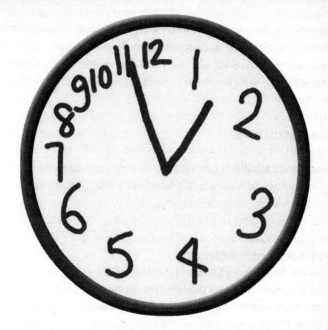

the diagnosis, the confirmation of dementia requires access to tests and facilities that are outside the scope of general practice. The impact and consequences of dementia are too great for there to be any doubt over its diagnosis. Primary care practitioners should be able to identify those people in whom dementia is reasonably likely and refer them for specialist assessment.

Specialist referral

Exactly what sort of specialist someone with dementia should first be seen by is not particularly important, provided the patient is ultimately directed to the right sorts of service and advice. Depending on the circumstances, someone with dementia might for example be seen by a psychiatrist or a specialist in the care of the elderly. Less commonly the specialist might be a physician in general medicine or a neurologist (specialist in diseases of the nervous system). Any and all of these specialists should be able to recognise dementia and put in train the necessary investigations to confirm it. Even more importantly they should be able to refer the patient and their carers to the right sort of support services, including voluntary ones, which can provide extra help to the patient and his or her family.

Memory clinics

One of the innovations brought in to rationalise dementia care over the past few years has been the 'memory clinic'. These are hospital-based and managed under the direction of medical specialists with special training and expertise in caring for dementia. The teams usually also include nurses, psychologists and other therapists with appropriate special experience.

One of the driving factors for the establishment of these clinics was the arrival of drug therapy for dementia in the late 1990s. Perhaps concerned that the medication would be over-prescribed and given to the wrong patients by GPs under pressure from anxious patients, or more especially their relatives, the UK government restricted the initiation of dementia drug treatment to specialists. GPs could continue the prescription of the drugs if they were happy to do so (not all are).

Memory clinics are one way of providing a more efficient service, by bringing all the relevant personnel under one roof, but their results have been mixed. They are not in place uniformly across the country and some have even closed under the pressure of too many referrals combined with inadequate funding. Exactly what any person's experience of dementia assessment and diagnosis is in the UK is still, therefore, too variable to generalise upon.

Assessment process

Whatever the local arrangements for dementia assessment are the basic principles are the same: to detect conditions other than dementia if present, to categorise the type of dementia as exactly as possible and to recommend the best treatment for the individual patient.

The first stages of the assessment can be mostly carried out by the GP. He or she has the patient's main medical records, knows what medication the patient is taking, often knows the family and what effects someone's dementia is beginning to have on them and in the long term will provide continuity of care along with the other members of the primary care team.

GP ASSESSMENT

Even when the GP knows a patient well the details of the symptoms as they have developed over the preceding months is of great value, in particular the observations of family and friends. The GP will look for clues to other conditions such as depression, some by using diagnostic questionnaires like those referred to earlier, but others working in a more intuitive way. There is no right or wrong way provided it gets the right answers! Often it will take more than one visit or consultation to carry out these assessments.

Examination of the patient, although good practice, will only rarely reveal some other medical condition. The value of a medical examination is therefore more often that it is negative than positive. Without going into excessive medical detail here it is nonetheless a valuable part of the process of diagnosis. Other points the doctor is looking for are elevation of the blood pressure, and whether the person smokes or has signs of poor circulation. If present these would raise the chance that atherosclerosis is contributing to the condition.

Blood tests for a range of major conditions such as diabetes, thyroid disease and kidney problems that can cause or contribute to confusion or dementia are done. At the same time a check can be made of the cholesterol level in the blood if it is not already known and the patient is not very elderly.

By the time this initial assessment by the primary care team is complete it is likely that a diagnosis of dementia can be reached with a high degree of certainty.

SPECIALIST ASSESSMENT

Even if the GP's work-up has covered all the essentials and it seems likely that the diagnosis of dementia is correct the specialist clinic is valuable from several aspects:

- confirming the diagnosis
- providing extra information to the patient and carers
- advising on treatment
- co-ordinating care
- follow-up

Confirming the diagnosis

Dementia is a permanent condition that can have a dramatic impact on an individual and his or her family, friends and other relationships. It is reasonable that the diagnosis should be made with the best achievable accuracy and that all reasonable attempts are made to diagnose alternative conditions that might masquerade as dementia. It follows that one of the functions of the specialist clinic is to arrange those investigations that are outside the scope of the GP team.

BRAIN SCANS

Brain scanning technology has moved on quite rapidly in the past few years and there are now several ways of imaging the brain. The important point is to ensure that brain tumours or other physical conditions that may need treatment in their own right are detected. CT scanning, which is a sophisticated type of X-ray picture that also uses computer technology to produce the image, is the basic test that can do this.

Despite their usefulness the UK still needs more scanners of this type to service the needs of modern medical investigation. Because access to scanning time is limited some doctors doubt the need for everyone presenting with dementia to have a brain scan but most take the view that it is too important in establishing the diagnosis with certainty to miss this test out.

There are other, newer, types of brain scan available, which in research studies are beginning to show details such as the region of the brain that is active. As yet the practical applications of these more sophisticated tests is unclear. The CT scan provides enough information to detect those conditions that might require separate action in someone with apparent dementia.

Specialised tests

LUMBAR PUNCTURE

In some parts of the world, but not routinely in the UK, examination of a sample of the fluid from around the brain is used as part of the investigation of someone with dementia. This clear fluid, called the cerebrospinal fluid (CSF), cushions the brain within the skull and extends down the length of the spinal canal, surrounding the spinal cord. It is possible to take a sample from it through a hypodermic needle inserted into the lower back, in a test called a lumbar puncture. Examination of the CSF in Alzheimer's disease shows elevated levels of tau protein as well as other recognisable changes. At present the value of CSF testing in diagnosis is uncertain but there is research interest in developing it so that it may become useful in the early detection of Alzheimer's disease.

ELECTRICAL ACTIVITY (BRAIN WAVES)

The electroencephalogram (EEG) is a recording of the electrical activity of the brain made by attaching a number of electrodes to the scalp. Some patterns in brain wave activity have been described in the different types of dementia but the main use of this test is in detecting rarer types of dementia, such as Creutzfeldt-Jakob disease (CJD) in which characteristic patterns of brain activity are seen.

Test for a reason

Common sense as well as clinical judgement are needed in deciding when to put people through specialised tests, or even the simpler ones. CT scanning is not easy to do in a frail elderly person who is unable to understand the procedure and co-operate with the need to lie down on the scanner table and keep still for some minutes, but it is well tolerated by those with early dementia. Lumbar puncture is not commonly done in the UK for dementia but in any case it is an invasive procedure and there may be ethical issues in obtaining informed consent from a patient to agree to such a test. In some parts of the world where access to technical investigations is easy there is a tendency to use every available test as a matter of routine. British doctors, in part through necessity, have a deserved reputation for being more selective in how they use technology to assess their patients.

Although it is important to achieve an accurate diagnosis this has to be done always with the purpose of helping the patient. Sometimes other medical circumstances will mean that a test result will make no difference to the person's treatment. In those circumstances the test cannot be justified.

Informing the patient and the carers

There is now a large amount of high quality information available to inform people about dementia and its consequences. The specialist clinic should ensure that this is made available, if this has not already been done by the GP team. The Alzheimer's Society is the largest charity devoted to dementia in the UK and it produces a wide range of high quality information for patients and carers both in print form and via its website (www.alzheimers.org.uk, see also appendix C). Many localities have also produced their own summaries of information concerning dementia, the services available for patients and carers in that region and how to access them.

Advising on treatment

Details on the drugs available for dementia follow in the next chapter. Normally the specialist recommends the treatment to the GP, who prescribes it under a 'shared-care' arrangement. Such schemes are the norm in most parts of the country but there may be places where they do not exist, or in which a particular GP practice is unhappy to participate in shared care. In those cases the patients will need to obtain their ongoing prescriptions from the specialist clinic.

Co-ordinating care

Again there may be differences in how this is arranged in different regions but the most effective dementia services ensure that all agencies that might need to be involved in an individual's care, from social services to consultant medical intervention, have a point of contact via the clinic. The patients and the carers then know what help they can expect from various agencies, and who the contact persons are for each of them.

Follow-up

The need for specialist follow-up can depend on whether drug therapy for dementia has been prescribed. The decision to continue such drugs depends largely on whether they appear to have had any effect, as well as on local arrangements for drug prescribing. Most such arrangements will tend to follow the general advice outlined by the National Institute for Clinical Excellence (NICE). NICE guidance is that the carer's view of the condition should be sought before and during drug treatment but also that the patient should be assessed initially between two and four months after drug treatment is established and thereafter at six-month intervals. However, after a while, testing every six months simply makes the patient distressed and adds nothing to the overall management, so in practice specialists make more informed individual decisions on the continuance of treatment.

Present dementia care arrangements

If the drug treatments available for dementia were very cheap it is debatable whether they would have attracted the attention of the National Institute for Clinical Excellence. The MMSE was never designed to be a tool that can be used repeatedly to gauge the effectiveness of dementia treatment, yet NICE has dictated that it should be used in this way. As far as we know the effect of dementia treatments cannot be monitored in a valid way using such simple tools, and even people who by NICE criteria have not 'improved' may still be benefiting from dementia drug therapy. There is, for example, a lot of supportive evidence to show that people on such drugs have a lower rate of eventually needing more specialist or hospital care. They may not show any improvement on their MMSE test but they may also have been saved from further deterioration, which is more difficult to prove but still worth achieving.

The presently available drugs for dementia offer limited benefits for people with dementia but they are the best we have. In the next chapter we consider them in more detail.

Chapter 6

Treatments for dementia

Drug treatments

In chapter 2 one of the topics covered was how neurotransmitter substances are involved in transmitting signals from one nerve cell to the next. To understand how the main drugs available for Alzheimer's disease work a little more detail of this process is required.

Neurotransmitters and drug action

Each time an amount of neurotransmitter substance is released from one cell and crosses the gap to the next then a signal is passed on. After a few such signals there would logically be a build-up of the neurotransmitter substance at the synapse. The signalling system would then break down as there would be so much neurotransmitter substance within the synapse that new signals would not be noticed. Nature has of course devised an ingenious way of dealing with this problem.

This takes the form of enzymes (which are proteins capable of speeding up a chemical reaction) present within the synapse gap, which destroy excess neurotransmitter molecules. If the nerve signal is likened to a message chalked on a blackboard this enzyme is the cleaning cloth that wipes the board clean as soon as the message is read. We previously mentioned that one of the main neuro-transmitters in the brain is acetyl choline. The enzyme that mops up excess acetyl choline in the course of normal nerve activity is called 'acetylcholinesterase', or just 'cholinesterase'.

You may recall that in Alzheimer's disease certain brain regions such as the hippocampi show marked loss of neurones and that these regions use acetyl choline as their main neurotransmitter. This loss of nerve signal 'traffic' in the affected regions is the main explanation we presently have for the symptoms of Alzheimer's disease. Drugs have been developed that reduce the activity of this enzyme, which therefore slows down the rate at which it destroys free acetyl choline. This has the effect of boosting the nerve signals produced by the smaller number of neurones still active in the brain of someone with Alzheimer's disease. To go back to our earlier analogy these drugs allow the message to stay on the board for a longer time before it is wiped off. The general term for these drugs is 'cholinesterase inhibitors'.

Cholinesterase inhibitors

These are the main drugs with beneficial activity in Alzheimer's disease. They are fairly new, first appearing for use in patients in the late 1990s. There are now three drugs in this group licensed for use in the UK (the drug's formal name is listed first and the manufacturer's brand name is in brackets):

1 Donepezil (Aricept®)

2 Galantamine (Reminyl®)
3 Rivastigmine (Exelon®)

There are some differences in the exact details of how these drugs work, but it is not very important to know them. More important in practical terms are that they all have potential side effects that can limit their use in some patients. These stem from the fact that the way nerve cells work applies to the whole nervous system and not just the brain. Acetyl choline is used widely as a neurotransmitter in nerves throughout the body. For example, it is used by some of the nerves that control the pulse rate of the heart, the width of the airways within the lungs, the activity of the muscles of the bowel and of the muscle that normally holds the outlet of the bladder closed. Increasing the activity of all these nerves slows the heart rate, tightens the airways, causes diarrhoea and makes it easier to pass urine. Sometimes the urine flows too easily, leading to incontinence.

Fortunately the drugs are designed to have relatively little of these undesirable effects but they cannot be avoided altogether. Additionally they can cause digestive upset, sleeplessness, headaches and other symptoms and they have to be used with caution in people with impaired kidney function, lung conditions such as asthma and some heart conditions. People with Parkinson's disease may find some of their symptoms get worse if they also have dementia and are given a cholinesterase inhibitor, so they may not be suitable for treatment with them. As with all drugs the list of possible side effects is quite off-putting but in practice these medicines are usually tolerated quite well.

Research trials in dementia

Very many research papers have now been published on the effects of these and other drugs in dementia. Such research is difficult to do for many reasons. Measuring 'quality of life' or 'functional ability' is more difficult than measuring blood pressure or body weight, where a machine tells you the right answer in seconds. In dementia the assessment tool is often a questionnaire or a survey, which is subject to more variation in results depending on how it is used. Often it is the opinion of a third party such as a carer that is recorded, rather than direct assessment of the patient. Dementia progresses relatively slowly, therefore observations of the effect of treatment have to be made over a long period of time. Many studies use time scales of only a few months, which makes it difficult to draw conclusions that apply to the long term. Often people in the age group most likely to have dementia have other medical problems that can alter the outcome of treatment in ways that do not necessarily relate directly to the dementia drugs. These are only some of the practical problems that come into play but as a result the research evidence for and against many types of treatment is not so solid as it is for other, more easily researched, conditions like high blood pressure or heart attacks. Almost all of the main research on drug treatment for dementia is in fact to do with Alzheimer's disease rather than the other types.

Results of cholinesterase inhibitor drugs in dementia

The first drug of this type, called tacrine, was associated with significant side effects and is no longer used in the UK. Donepezil, rivastigmine and galantamine are 'second-generation' cholinesterase inhibitors and all improve intellectual function ('cognitive function') compared to dummy treatment (placebo) in trials over periods of up to around 12 months.

- One large research trial showed that donepezil delayed the average rate of decline in people treated with it by about five months.
- Rivastigmine is the only cholinesterase inhibitor shown so far to improve symptoms in Lewy body dementia. It is also effective in Alzheimer's disease and may be more effective in those people

who also have raised blood pressure or other risk factors for vascular disease. Side effects such as nausea, vomiting and reduced appetite were common with rivastigmine in these studies.

- Galantamine improved cognitive function and overall clinical state over six months compared to placebo in people with Alzheimer's disease or vascular dementia. Higher doses are more effective and increasing the dose slowly improves the tolerance to the drug.

Not much research comparing the cholinesterase inhibitors against each other has yet been done. Although they may seem to have different effects in different types of dementia this is more likely to reflect the nature of the research studies in which they have been used. There is no evidence that combining the different cholinesterase inhibitors is of any additional value but it may be worth trying more than one in sequence, especially if there are problems with side effects from the first chosen.

The question of how long to use these drugs is open to debate. Even if they do not cause obvious improvement they may help to slow the progress of dementia in an individual, but that benefit is impossible to measure. NICE guidance does not set any upper limit and makes it clear that if there is an impression that the drug is working then provided there are no problems with it, it should be continued. Many experts believe that once the decision is made to prescribe a cholinesterase inhibitor it should be considered a permanent treatment.

AD2000 STUDY

At the time of writing (July 2004) a study, called the AD2000 study, into the effects of donepezil has been published in the *Lancet* that casts doubt on the effectiveness of this drug (see appendix A for reference). This study recruited 565 patients with Alzheimer's disease, with or without associated vascular dementia, and observed the effects of donepezil compared with placebo (dummy treatment).

In addition to the patients' performance on tests of cognitive function other measures of effectiveness of the treatment were the time it took for anyone in the trial to deteriorate to the extent of needing institutional care or to show significant impairment in functional ability.

The study confirmed that donepezil produced small improvements in cognitive function and in the ability to carry out the activities of daily living in people with mild to moderate Alzheimer's disease. However, the study failed to show any effect of donepezil in slowing the rate at which people with Alzheimer's disease deteriorated enough to need institutionalised care, or in the progress of significant disability.

Critics of this study have already pointed out that it recruited a small number of patients – perhaps not enough to show benefits, and there were other reasons that might have muddied the results. The debate will undoubtedly go on concerning the effectiveness of cholinesterase inhibitors. There are certainly many advocates for their use among the world-wide body of experts in dementia, but they are not by any means wonder drugs. Only about half of those started on treatment show good response, but it is not clear what the differences are between those who respond and those who don't.

Memantine (Ebixa®)

Other nerve and neurotransmitter reactions exist in addition to those previously described and appear to be relevant to dementia. One of these other neurotransmitters is a substance called glutamate. The key action of glutamate is that it increases neurone activity. One of the other theories that has been put forward to explain Alzheimer's disease is that there is over-activity of the glutamate system. Memantine is a drug that partially blocks the action of glutamate, thus dampening down this over-activity. Memantine is licensed for use in moderate to severe Alzheimer's disease. Studies on small numbers of patients show that it has a small effect but the exact role of this drug is still unclear.

Vascular dementia

In people whose dementia is purely vascular in type cholinesterase inhibitors and memantine have not been shown to be effective. As many people have 'mixed' dementia in which Alzheimer's disease and vascular dementia co-exist they can possibly benefit from these drugs. Additionally, people who have significant risk factors present for developing atherosclerosis, such as high blood pressure or high cholesterol levels, or who smoke, can benefit both in their general health and in the rate of progress of their dementia by having these risk factors treated.

STATIN TREATMENT

'Statins' refer to a group of drugs that are now the most widely used in lowering raised levels of cholesterol in the blood. There is an expanding amount of medical research to support the idea that statins might slow the rate of development of Alzheimer's disease. Statins are already known to significantly reduce the risk of problems arising from atherosclerosis, particularly in people with diabetes. Although more research is needed to clarify the exact role of statins in dementia they should be seriously considered in anyone who is at above average risk for having or developing vascular disease.

Gingko biloba

This extract of the leaves of the maidenhair tree has a long history of use as a traditional remedy for a range of diseases. It is widely prescribed in Europe for problems such as confusion, memory impairment, anxiety and headaches. It can be bought in the UK without prescription. Some small studies have shown a positive effect on cognitive function but more recent studies have given inconsistent results. Until larger studies are done the evidence is inconclusive. Gingko biloba is safe and has no significant side effects but it may interact with other drugs and reduce their effectiveness, or increase their side effects.

One of the difficulties with traditional products is the variability in the amount of active product within different preparations. It may take as much as a year of regular use before any benefit is seen.

Drugs with uncertain or no proven benefit

VITAMIN E

Vitamin E is a powerful antioxidant and therefore capable of mopping up the 'free radical' molecules derived from oxygen that are possibly implicated in cell ageing and dementia. Taking the results of various research studies together indicates no benefit in cognitive function from two years' of vitamin E supplements but a possibly beneficial effect on reducing long-term deterioration in Alzheimer's disease.

OTHER DRUGS

As mentioned in chapter 3, earlier studies suggesting possible benefit from non-steroidal anti-inflammatory drugs and hormone replacement therapy have not been confirmed and neither is now recommended in dementia.

Non-drug treatments

There is naturally much interest in treatments that do not rely on drug therapy, which as we've just seen is by no means very effective in many people with dementia. Unfortunately the medical literature again suffers here from a lack of good quality, long-term studies involving lots of patients. Several types of non-drug treatment exist and the amount of evidence in favour of each varies from a lot to very little.

STIMULATION

People who in their youth have had a higher level of education or have been throughout their lives involved in repeated learning situations show less tendency to have memory problems when they get older. Using your brain seems to keep it more active for longer. A brief trip around some residential establishments for people with severe dementia will quickly show that stimulation is not something that many of them get a great deal of. Treatments along the lines of helping someone with dementia to interact more with their environment and with other people have been shown to improve their scores on cognitive function and to improve their quality of life.

Using reminiscences can help someone engage in topics and these memories can be used to relate to present day living. Quizzes, card games, crosswords, reading, music and aromatherapy are all ways of stimulating the various senses. Individual studies looking at the effects of music therapy or reminiscence therapy alone do not show clear results, as much because of the difficulties of studying their effects in isolation as anything else, but trials of 'multisensory stimulation' show more positive results (for some people, during the sessions only). Such programmes are, however, demanding of time from carers and they need to be carried out repeatedly for the benefits to be sustained.

To someone affected by dementia the activities of daily living that ordinarily seem mundane become more important. Bathing, dressing and other self-care tasks may need to be helped (for example, someone might be unable to find the toothbrush but if it is first placed in his hand he can use it). Actions like setting the table, washing the windows or baking a cake may be familiar from the past and are therefore more likely to be still within someone's repertoire even if they have quite marked dementia.

SNOEZELEN

Snoezelen is a type of multi-sensory therapy developed originally in Holland for people with learning disability. The word comes from two Dutch ones – 'snuffelen' (to seek out or explore) and 'doezelen' (to relax). The therapy involves rooms with lots of different types of stimulation in the form of light, sound, smell and touch. Snoezelen has become quite widely used in educational and care settings for children with special educational needs such as autism. There is some research evidence on the effect of snoezelen therapy in dementia but not enough to reach any conclusions. Other studies are under way to clarify this.

CARER TRAINING AND SUPPORT

Education of carers in what to expect in dementia and how to handle a person who has the condition significantly improves the outcome both for the patient, who is less likely to need institutional care, and for the carer who feels more able to cope. Caring for someone with dementia can be very hard work, not to say completely exhausting, and no matter how much the person with dementia is loved, their behaviour can still be very trying. People caring for others with dementia are more likely than average to experience anxiety and depression themselves. More on the topic of 'caring for the carers' is contained in chapter 9.

REALITY ORIENTATION

Dementia commonly causes disorientation, which in turn can cause insecurity and anxiety in the person with dementia. Reality orientation originated in rehabilitation work with war veterans and was adapted as a technique to improve the quality of life of confused elderly people. Reality orientation includes repeatedly but informally confirming to the person where they are, what the day and date is and what it is that they are doing. There is some evidence that reality orientation has benefits for mental function and behaviour in people with dementia. Disadvantages include possible lowering of self-esteem and mood from the constant re-learning of the same material.

BRIGHT LIGHT THERAPY

Sleep disturbance caused by dementia can be particularly upsetting for carers already tired out and needing rest. Using bright light therapy to change the person's biological clock back towards 'normal' is labour intensive and unfortunately the published evidence on this type of treatment is of poor quality. There is presently insufficient evidence to make any recommendation on the merits of this treatment.

BEHAVIOUR THERAPY

This can use a reward system that encourages desired behaviour. It can be used to try and change unwanted behaviour such as aggression or wandering. Although some success has been reported, not everyone responds and the improvement can be quite short-lived.

VALIDATION THERAPY

This accepts the patient's view of reality so that interaction causes them less distress. Validation therapy has been criticised by researchers. The available evidence says it is ineffective.

COMPLEMENTARY THERAPY

There has been a tremendous increase in the popularity and use of 'complementary' medical therapies in the past 10 to 15 years. In part this is perhaps a reaction against what many see as the over-reliance of Western medicine on prescribing a pill for every ill. It also reflects a growing need for people to take more active control over their medical care. The range of treatments that fall under the description of complementary treatments is huge – there are literally hundreds of different types of treatment. Some, such as homoeopathy and acupuncture, have become more widely accepted by conventional medicine in recent years – in fact homoeopathy has always been available as a prescribable treatment since the NHS was formed in 1948.

Research studies on complementary therapies all tend to suffer from the same problems of small scale and, often, poor study design. As a result any benefits, or harms, are hard to define. Medical research is very expensive and most of the money that goes into research comes from pharmaceutical companies investigating the effects of their products. A good study showing positive results in favour of a drug will potentially be worth huge sums to a drug company. In contrast complementary treatments are not usually worth large sums of money. Often they are not patented and cannot be capitalised on. The fact that so few complementary therapies show any effects in dementia partly reflects this problem with getting good quality research studies done.

Consequently it is not possible to make any definite recommendations on what type of treatment to choose, but this does not mean that they are not worth trying. Aromatherapy, herbal medicine, homoeopathy, acupuncture and music therapy are probably the most commonly used, but they can also have their own sorts of side effects and some people do not tolerate these sorts of treatment.

CONCLUSIONS

Treatment for dementia, whether drug-based or non-drug based, needs to be tailored to the individual. Often more than one approach is needed simultaneously. The medicines we presently have available can give benefit to many patients in the right circumstances. For example cholinesterase inhibitors are better for mild dementia when behavioural problems are not severe, whereas 'antipsychotic' drugs can help control severe behavioural problems. Non-drug approaches have the advantage of being safe and also allow some degree of self-empowerment in tackling the illness.

Other help

There is a great deal of help available to someone with dementia and to his or her carers and the best use should be made of it. The GP can advise on general aspects of care and medical treatment as well as liaise with most of the other professionals that might be involved. The district nurse can talk more knowledgeably about the practical aspects of daily care, such as bathing and washing. When necessary, aids such as bath hoists and stair lifts can be provided for people with impaired mobility. Usually these will be provided free or are grant-aided. Other practical measures that can help improve the home environment are the province of the occupational therapist, who can come to the house and make an assessment. Physiotherapists can advise on maintaining flexibility and fitness or on exercises that are appropriate for someone with a disability.

The local social security office and Citizen's Advice service can be consulted on applying for the right benefits, including attendance allowance for carer expenses. People with any chronic disability, including dementia, are entitled to an assessment of their needs by the social work department. Ultimately people who need long-term care are entitled to have funding for it, depending on their financial circumstances, and the social work department or local authority office can advise on this.

Voluntary organisations such as the Alzheimer's Society have branches across the country as well as their Helpline and website containing many helpful factsheets. Local support groups, especially those specifically aimed at dementia sufferers and their carers, can provide practical help and advice based on shared experiences.

Someone with dementia will probably need help with managing their financial affairs and legal advice may be needed on this. 'Enduring power of attorney' (called 'continuing power of attorney'

67

in Scotland) is a means of enabling another person to take command of an individual's affairs should he become incapable of doing so for himself later in life. Welfare power of attorney enables someone to take decisions on a person's care and treatment, should they need it. Making these appointments before a person loses capacity can save a great deal of trouble later on.

All of these areas are as much a part of the treatment of dementia as any prescription medicine, and are often far more important.

People with dementia, as well as their carers, need help to deal with the illness. They need to learn what to expect as time goes by as far as the effects of the dementia are concerned and they need practical tips on how to cope. Much of this information is now provided in the form of carer support information and through the personal input of those staff trained to provide it. Despite the regional variations in provision of dementia care referred to earlier no part of the UK is without access to good quality support and advice, so make sure you ask for it.

Chapter 7

General principles of dementia care

What is most useful in dementia care is not which drug to take (as their benefits are limited) but how to manage day-to-day living with the condition. You can't push dementia away or hide it with medicines, so you have to get on with it. (The following information is partly abridged from the Department of Health's excellent publication *Who Cares* – details of which are in appendix A.)

Maintain dignity

People with dementia are not stupid, nor do they revert to being children or become suddenly deaf. Many people who haven't taken the time to learn about dementia behave towards someone with dementia as if all of these features applied. Particularly in the earlier phases of the illness the affected person will still retain much of their intellectual capacity. They will appreciate being treated with respect and not talked down to. Even when dementia progresses and someone's ability to look after themselves is impaired they still deserve to be given their dignity.

Keep things normal

If you had a routine or a hobby or pastime that you shared, keep it going. Perhaps it will become harder to maintain a complete sense of normality and ultimately it might become impossible to do certain activities requiring concentration, memory or co-ordination but the longer these activities can be kept going the better. By the same token it is important to let someone keep doing things that maintain their independence until they become unable to cope. They may get a lot slower at it but provided they are managing and not finding it stressful then it is therapeutic for them and keeps your workload lower too.

Avoid confrontation

Disagreements can arise when what the person with dementia thinks is sensible behaviour conflicts with what most other people would think. For example, going out in the rain only in pyjamas, or flushing money down the toilet. Telling someone with dementia that they are wrong doesn't work and may make matters worse. Instead it is better to distract them, guiding them away from any potential trouble. They will probably forget about the undesirable behaviour soon enough anyway.

Plan ahead

A crisis to someone with dementia could be being hurried to do something that they are not prepared for or when going into unfamiliar surroundings. Any sort of change can be difficult for someone with dementia to cope with, and it is impossible to avoid change in life. Whenever possible though, try to anticipate new events well ahead. In new situations try also to provide some continuity with the familiar, even if this is only your presence.

Routines help to maintain order and repetition helps someone with dementia to remain oriented and avoid becoming bewildered.

Keep it simple

Giving someone with dementia too many things to do at once will increase their level of anxiety and may cause them to become fearful or flustered. Tasks need to be broken down into their component parts and taken one or two steps at a time.

Keep it safe

The ordinary household can be a dangerous place for someone who is getting less steady on their feet and easily gets lost going from one room to the next. Gas fires and cookers are obvious potential hazards. An occupational therapist can help check your house and advise on things you can do to make it safer.

Keep healthy

Everyone needs to keep active and eat healthily, and people with dementia are no exception. Until such time as it becomes impractical it is good to get the person out for a walk or do some other form of appropriate exercise. There is no diet that is specifically beneficial for dementia but adaptation of the diet may become necessary if the person has difficulty feeding themselves for any reason.

Keep communicating

Dementia can affect someone's ability to use language. They may use the wrong word and so be unable to say what they want to say. The person listening might be equally perplexed trying to work out what the message is. Both may end up becoming very frustrated. When communication difficulties start to become greater it is important to persevere and not give up trying to understand. Keep the conversation simple and don't talk about too many things at once. Be prepared to repeat things often if necessary. Remember that communication is not just about speech but includes non-verbal actions such as touch and body language.

Memory aids

Lots of little tricks to aid memory are useful in the earlier stages of dementia. For example:

- *Orientation*
  - O Keep furniture in the same place.
  - O Remind someone often of the time, day and where they are.
  - O Have pictures of familiar faces on display.
  - O Use memory aids such as labels, drawings or colours on doors to remind the person of where the bathroom is, and the bedroom etc.
- *Routines*
  - O Make up lists that can be referred to or checked off.
  - O Set things out in the order they need to be done.
  - O Use all the senses – sight, sound, touch, taste and smell in imaginative ways that can provide information.

Relax

If you are tense or hesitant when you are with someone with dementia they will pick it up and become more anxious. Try to engage someone with dementia just as you would a person of the same age without dementia. Find out how people like to deal with others. Touch, joviality and closeness suit some but not all.

Be prepared to experiment

If something you try doesn't work, don't dismiss it completely. Look for small changes and work on improving these. Carers have a lot of expertise, but sometimes they don't recognise it!

Chapter 8

Behavioural problems in dementia

Dementia does not only cause symptoms like memory loss and word-finding difficulty. A range of associated behavioural changes occurs, which can sometimes lead to more difficulties than the dementia symptoms. These include depression, agitation and aggression, wandering, sleep disturbance and more severe problems such as hallucinations. Doctors often use the term 'behavioural and psychological symptoms of dementia', or BPSD, in reference to these.

Depression

Depression affects up to 20 per cent of people with dementia and can be hard to detect, as symptoms such as slowness of thought or lack of interest are common to both conditions. As people with dementia commonly lack insight into what is happening to them they do not respond to non-drug types of treatment such as psychological therapy. Anti-depressant drug therapy is therefore the mainstay of treatment. Most of the newer anti-depressant drugs, such as fluoxetine (Prozac®) and its successors are suitable whereas the older anti-depressants (e.g. amitriptyline) are less so as they can interfere with the effects of cholinesterase inhibitor drugs, or cause problems of their own.

As with all drugs used in dementia, the person taking them may need help to remember to do so. In depression though, there may be considerable apathy, increasing the likelihood that doses will be missed out. If this is so then measures may be needed to make it easier to remember the daily drug schedule, which in turn may mean a family member or community nurse has to be involved.

Agitation and aggression

These problems arise in about half of all people with dementia. Related behaviour includes lack of inhibition (e.g. sexual), hyper-activity and confrontation. Often such behaviour is quite short-lived.

When behaviour changes abruptly the doctor needs to check that there is not a precipitating cause, such as a urine infection or some other potentially correctable illness. Unless such a cause is found then strategies to tackle the agitation without using drugs should be tried first. Structuring the person's day, avoiding them feeling rushed, confirming where they are and providing other reassurances may help defuse some of their anxiety.

Agitation is often fuelled by frustration, which in turn is worsened by disorientation and anxiety. One of the first tactics is to counter this with reassurance and support. For example, someone with dementia might become increasingly agitated about being unable to remember something. They may repeat the same question and get the same answer but increasingly become frustrated at needing to be reminded of the information. In turn you might become tired of having to repeat the same information, and this might come out in your tone of voice, if not more directly. Instead of repeating your answer it might be better to break the cycle, say by hugging your partner and reminding him that everything is fine and that he is safe where he is, etc.

DRUG TREATMENT

When someone becomes increasingly agitated and potentially or actively aggressive, when one is sure this is not secondary to some other correctable cause and when simpler techniques for defusing the situation have not worked, drug treatment may need to be used. Several drugs within the groups known as tranquillisers or anti-psychotics have been tried in this situation. The best researched is haloperidol, which is effective but is also associated with a high frequency of side effects such as muscle stiffness and involuntary movements.

Newer drugs such as risperidone and olanzapine are capable of reducing aggression and until March 2004 had been increasingly used to manage behavioural and psychological symptoms in dementia, although neither drug had a product licence to be used in this way. However, the Committee on Safety of Medicines (CSM), which is the monitoring and advisory body in the UK on the use of drugs, released guidance in March 2004 that doctors should no longer prescribe these drugs to people with dementia. For reasons that are unclear these drugs put people with dementia at increased risk of subsequently having a stroke compared with placebo treatment. This risk was seen in patients with all types of dementia and not just those with the vascular type.

Several other drugs have been used in controlling the behavioural and psychological symptoms of dementia to some extent. Some examples are carbamazepine and sodium valproate, which are anti-epileptic drugs, and trazodone, which is a type of anti-depressant.

The cholinesterase inhibitors donepezil and galantamine, apart from their effects on the direct symptoms of Alzheimer's disease, may also have some beneficial effects on associated behavioural disturbance, although the evidence is weak.

Sleep disturbance

The carers of someone with dementia can put up with quite a bit if they at least get a decent sleep regularly but sleep disturbance is a common problem that accompanies dementia. If people frequently nap during the day they need less sleep at night, and daytime napping is one of the commonest causes of the problem. This can be made worse by sedative medicines that cause the patient to doze off during the day. When someone with dementia takes a daytime nap it may be seen as the carer's chance to catch up with the housework, but the consequence of night-time waking may be a poor trade-off.

Leaving someone in front of a television set is a sure way to have them nod off, so instead it is preferable to engage them in some sort of activity, whether it be craftwork or drying the dishes or going for walk. Short-term use of sleeping tablets can tide over a crisis but in the longer term they work less well.

Environmental lighting has an influence on sleep patterns and increased lighting in the afternoon and early evening hours may help to establish a more 'normal' rhythm.

Wandering

Many people with dementia go through a phase where they wander off. Often one can think of reasons why this should happen, such as disorientation after a move of house or relocation to a care home, or it may be secondary to forgetting the reason why they have set off on a journey in the first place or may reflect insecurity and a desire to find their carer if they have been left alone for a while.

Drug treatment for wandering is ineffective – all it can do is make the person so drowsy that they stay put, which apart from being inappropriate also increases their risk of having a fall. Locking a person in the house to prevent wandering is of doubtful legality and can be potentially dangerous. It is better to alert neighbours and maybe the local shops and ask them to let you know should the person show up on their premises looking lost. Identification labels inside clothes or some other means of identification are useful. Most people with dementia who wander do not end up getting into much trouble, despite all the anxiety they might cause.

Delusions and hallucinations

A delusion is a false, fixed belief and a hallucination is a false perception of something that is not there. Hallucinations are usually either of sound or vision but they can be of smell or taste.

Common delusions in dementia are variations on the theme of persecution. The person may, for example, believe that people, including close family, are out to steal from them or carry out some other form of mischief such as poisoning their food. Hallucinations are real to the person experiencing them so they might be reassuring or be frightening and provoke more aggression.

As with agitation, the doctor needs to be sure there is not some other underlying cause for the behaviour that he can deal with. The appropriate management of delusions and hallucinations depends more on their consequences than their presence. If non-threatening, the patient and the carers may not need any action except understanding on the part of the people around. If more disturbed behaviour needs to be treated with drugs then haloperidol is a common choice, starting with a small dose to minimise side effects and working up to the required dose. Where hallucinations are visual and especially if associated with dementia with Lewy bodies, cholinesterase inhibitors can be quite helpful. Behavioural and psychological management in dementia is a specialised field and the GP will usually call upon the help of a specialist for advice, such as an Old Age Psychiatrist.

Chapter 9

Caring for the carers

Emotions

Caring for a loved one who has developed dementia is an emotional roller coaster. At times it is sad, at other times it can be funny. It is usually hard work and can often cause many conflicting feelings, amongst them guilt, anger and frustration but hopefully also a sense of achievement and pride at times. Relationships are often imperfect, even when both partners are in good health, and one partner becoming unwell doesn't mean that problems sort themselves out.

ANGER AND GUILT

In many ways the emotions that a carer goes through are similar to those when someone dies. Initially learning that your partner, say, has dementia may provoke feelings of anger – why me? Why us?

You may become frustrated at delays in getting tests done to confirm what is wrong or become antagonistic to the diagnosis, looking for a second opinion. The realities of what is available for the treatment of the condition will seem inadequate as most offer only modest improvements in some aspects of the condition and there are certainly no cures.

Some of that anger might be directed at the medical profession but some of it will also be aimed at the person who has the dementia. You might assume prematurely that your life with your partner is effectively over or you might worry that they will deteriorate quickly and soon need institutional care. The nature of your early thoughts about dementia are likely, therefore, to be overwhelmingly negative.

Guilt may come because you worry that you are not doing enough to help the person with dementia or because you didn't sort out relationship problems in the past, or it may come later if a move to residential care becomes necessary. The latter may come very close to the experience of losing the person as if they had died.

FRUSTRATION AND RESENTMENT

The initial need in dementia is to have the diagnosis confirmed accurately, and we've seen earlier what that process entails. Waiting lists for dementia clinics are probably always going to be longer than anyone wishes, so the weeks or months waiting for an appointment are going to drag very slowly. On the one hand you may be reluctant to have the diagnosis made official, because there's no going back from dementia. On the other hand having the diagnosis confirmed is a relief as it validates the symptoms, allows access to treatment and let's you plan for the future.

Many of the things that someone with dementia will say and do can be hard to bear, or even be directly hurtful. When someone you might have lived with for most of your adult life shows no sign of recognition in looking at your face it is not easy to take. When they become physically aggressive, or accuse you of stealing from them, you may well become resentful or respond in kind.

Get help early

Most people with dementia will wish to live in their own home for as long as possible, and the same goes for their partners. At an early stage it is best to ask for help or at least be sure of what help is available, and how you can access it. Your GP, or the GP looking after the person with dementia, should be able to put you in touch with all of the services mentioned earlier as well as give you the contact details for at least the main voluntary organisations such as the Alzheimer's Society.

Check that you are claiming all the benefits that you are entitled to and if you are uncertain which ones you should have then ask at your social security office or Citizen's Advice Bureau. Often the practice nurse or health visitor at the GP's surgery is also well able to advise on what you should be claiming for and can help you fill out the forms too if need be.

Look after yourself

Your own health, both mental and physical, is going to be all the more important as your role as carer becomes more prominent over the years, so it is wise to ask your doctor for a check-up. Depression and anxiety are more common in carers of people with dementia than in the average population. Having a dependent partner does not make you immune from having your own health needs. If your GP is not the same doctor who is caring for the person with dementia make sure that you tell them what your home circumstances are. GPs know the system in their area, what sorts of service are available and who the right people are to get things organised, so ask to be put in touch with these personnel.

You can't get too much information about dementia or get it too soon, so even if you think you know enough about it, or if you feel you are managing just fine at the moment and don't need any help, make that contact sooner rather than later.

TAKE BREAKS

One of the most important parts of caring is not caring – i.e. you need to get a break from it regularly. This could be when a volunteer comes into the house for a couple of hours once a week to let you get to the shops or have a coffee with a friend, or it might mean that your partner goes into respite care for a few weeks every now and then to let you have a bigger break. Every part of the country has some facilities available to give carers respite breaks and you are entitled to have access to those facilities.

Day centres are another good way in which you can get some relief from always being on call and have some time for yourself. Usually they will also provide transport there and back for the patient.

If there is a perfect carer out there somewhere, who never loses their temper with their partner with dementia, who never harbours any feelings of resentment, anger or self-pity about what they have to cope with and who never feels guilty about wishing it had all turned out otherwise, then good luck to them, but they must be very few and far between. Most of us have to live with the fact that we are not perfect, and there is no shame in that.

Appendix A

References

Government and official publications

- National Service Framework for Older People: http://www.nhsia. nhs.uk/nsf/pages/published/olderpeople.asp?om=m1
- NHS, 'Who cares? Information and support for the carers of people with dementia': http://www.dh.gov.uk/assetRoot/04/08/ 23/74/04082374.pdf
- Committee on Safety of Medicines, 'Atypical antipsychotic drugs and stroke'; http://www.mca.gov.uk/ourwork/monitorsafe qualmed/safetymessages/antipsystroke_9304.htm
- National Institute for Clinical Excellence (NICE), 'Guidance on the use of drugs for Alzheimer's disease'; www.nice.org.uk/ page.aspx?o=14400

Review articles

- BMJ Publishing Group's Clinical Evidence, 'Dementia' (Clinical Evidence, 2004; 11: 1250–77); www.clinicalevidence.com/ceweb/conditions/index.jsp
- Royal College of Psychiatrists, 'Dementia at your fingertips'; www.rcpsych.ac.uk/college/faculty/dementia/index.htm
- Cochrane Dementia and Cognitive Improvement Group, 'Abstracts of Cochrane Reviews' (The Cochrane Library, Issue 3, 2004); www.update-software.com/abstracts/DEMENTIAAbstract Index.htm

Reviews in this include:

O antidepressants for treating depression in dementia
O aromatherapy for dementia
O aspirin for vascular dementia
O cholinesterase inhibitors for dementia with Lewy bodies
O cognitive rehabilitation and cognitive training for early-stage Alzheimer's disease and vascular dementia
O donepezil for dementia due to Alzheimer's disease
O donepezil for vascular cognitive impairment
O effect of the treatment of Type II diabetes mellitus on the development of cognitive impairment and dementia
O galantamine for dementia due to Alzheimer's disease
O ginkgo biloba for cognitive impairment and dementia
O haloperidol for agitation in dementia
O homeopathy for dementia
O hormone replacement therapy to maintain cognitive function in women with dementia
O ibuprofen for Alzheimer's disease
O lecithin for dementia and cognitive impairment
O light therapy for managing sleep, behaviour and mood disturbances in dementia
O memantine for dementia

- music therapy for people with dementia
- nicotine for Alzheimer's disease
- physostigmine for dementia due to Alzheimer's disease
- reality orientation for dementia
- reminiscence therapy for dementia
- respite care for people with dementia and their carers
- rivastigmine for Alzheimer's disease
- selegiline for Alzheimer's disease
- snoezelen for dementia
- statins for the prevention of Alzheimer's disease
- subjective barriers to prevent wandering of cognitively impaired people
- thiamine for Alzheimer's disease
- thioridazine for dementia
- transcutaneous electrical nerve stimulation (TENS) for dementia
- validation therapy for dementia
- valproic acid for agitation in dementia
- velnacrine for Alzheimer's disease
- vitamin E for Alzheimer's disease

Papers

- Lee, P. E. et al., 'Atypical antipsychotic drugs in the treatment of behavioural and psychological symptoms of dementia' (British Medical Journal, 2004; 329: 75–78); http://bmj.bmjjournals.com/cgi/content/full/329/7457/75
- AD 2000 Collaborative Group, 'Long-term donepezil treatment in 565 patients with Alzheimer's disease (AD2000): randomised double-blind trial' (The Lancet, 2004; 363: 2105–15); www.thelancet.com
- British Medical Journal's collected resources on dementia: http://bmj.bmjjournals.com/cgi/collection/dementia

Alzheimer's Society

The following factsheets are available from the Alzheimer's Society
or downloadable from their website, www.alzheimers.org.uk:

No.   *Title*
505   Activities (Jan 2000)
428   Adaptations, improvements and repairs to the home (Oct 2003)
509   Aggressive behaviour (Jan 2000)
446   Aids-related cognitive impairment (What is . . . ?) (Aug 2003)
406   Aluminium and Alzheimer's disease (Jun 2002)
401   Alzheimer's disease (What is . . . ?) (Jun 2003)
450   Am I at risk of developing Alzheimer's disease? (Oct 2001)
456   The brain and behaviour (Feb 2002)
410   Brain tissue donations (Jun 2002)
528   Care on general hospital ward (Oct 2000)
523   Carers – looking after yourself (Jan 2000)
465   Choices in care (March 2003)
427   CJD (What is . . . ?) (Aug 2003)
500   Communication (Jan 2000)
418   Community care assessment (Jan 2004)
434   Complementary and alternative medicine and dementia (Mar 2003)
414   Council tax (Aug 2003)
400   Dementia (What is . . . ?) (Jun 2003)
408   Dementia: drugs used to relieve behavioural symptoms (Mar 2004)
403   Dementia with Lewy bodies (What is . . . ?) (Aug 2003)
448   Dental care and dementia (Oct 2001)
444   Depression (Oct 2001)
426   Diagnosis and assessment (Nov 2000)
473   Direct payments (Mar 2004)
510   Dressing (Jan 2000)
527   Driving and dementia (Jan 2000)
407   Drug treatments for Alzheimer's disease – Aricept, Exelon, Reminyl and Ebixa (Aug 2003)

408 Drugs used to relieve behavioural symptoms (Mar 2004)

511 Eating (Jan 2000)

472 Enduring power of attorney (April 2003)

429 Equipment to help with disability (June 2003)

515 Explaining to children (Jan 2000)

516 Feelings of guilt (Jan 2000)

467 Financial and legal tips (April 2003)

404 Fronto-temporal dementia including Pick's disease (What is . . . ?) (Oct 2003)

464 Future medical treatment: advance statements (Sept 2002)

405 Genetics and dementia (June 2003)

460 Going on holiday (Aug 2002)

507 Grief and bereavement (Jan 2000)

520 Hallucinations and delusions (Jan 2000)

454 How health professionals can help (Dec 2001)

425 How the GP can help (Jan 2003)

502 Incontinence (July 2001)

438 Korsakoff's syndrome (What is . . . ?) (Jun 2003)

417 Later stages of dementia (May 2003)

430 Learning disabilities and dementia (Jan 2000)

517 Living alone (May 2003)

521 Maintaining skills (Jan 2000)

526 Memory loss in dementia (Jan 2000)

436 MMSE – a guide for people with dementia and their carers (Jun 2002)

471 Next steps (March 2003)

452 NHS-funded nursing care: the new assessments (Nov 2001)

468 Paying care home fees (April 2003)

404 Pick's disease and frontal lobe dementia (What is . . . ?) (Oct 2003)

512 Pressure sores (Jan 2000)

458 Progression of dementia (Jan 2002)

442 Rarer causes of dementia (Oct 2003)

503 Safety at home (Jan 2000)

532 Selecting a care home (Oct 2001)

514 Sexual difficulties (Jan 2000)

462 Short-term care (Aug 2002)

522 Staying healthy (Jan 2000)

474 Travelling (Jun 2004)

524 Understanding and respecting the person with dementia (Jan 2000)

525 Unusual behaviour (Jan 2000)

402 Vascular dementia (What is . . . ?) (Feb 2001)

409 Volunteering for research into dementia (Nov 2000)

501 Walking about or 'wandering' (Jan 2000)

504 Washing and bathing (Jan 2000)

413 Welfare benefits (Nov 2003)

518 What if I have dementia? (Jan 2000)

446 What is Aids-related cognitive impairment? (Aug 2003)

401 What is Alzheimer's disease? (Jun 2003)

427 What is CJD? (Aug 2003)

400 What is dementia? (Jun 2003)

403 What is dementia with Lewy bodies? (Aug 2003)

404 What is fronto-temporal dementia including Pick's disease? (Oct 2003)

438 What is Korsakoff's syndrome? (Jun 2003)

402 What is vascular dementia? (Feb 2001)

440 Younger people with dementia (Jul 2001)

The Alzheimer's Society also has the following tests on its website:

- Mini Mental State Examination (MMSE):
  www.alzheimers.org.uk/Working_with_people_with_dementia/Primary_care/Dementia_diagnosis_and_management_in_primary_care/mmse.html
- Carer Strain Index:
  www.alzheimers.org.uk/Working_with_people_with_dementia/Primary_care/Dementia_diagnosis_and_management_in_primary_care/csi.html

Appendix B

Drugs

The following information contains selected details of some of the medications used in treating dementia. Full details are included in the manufacturer's data sheets and can also be viewed within the medicines section of the NetDoctor website: http://www.netdoctor.co.uk/medicines/

The information is accurate at the time of writing but new information on medicines appears regularly. A health professional should always be consulted concerning the prescription and use of medicines.

Medicines and their possible side effects can affect individual people in different ways. The following lists some of the side effects that are known to be associated with these medicines. Side effects other than those listed may exist.

Anticholinesterases

Donepezil, galantamine and rivastigmine are the three main drugs used in the treatment of Alzheimer's disease and are classified as anticholinesterases. This means that they inhibit the action of the enzyme acetylcholinesterase. Acetylcholine is a neurotransmitter substance used in the brain and nervous system, and reduced levels of acetylcholine in certain parts of the brain is a feature of Alzheimer's disease. The action of these drugs has the effect of boosting the effect of the available acetylcholine, which can lead to an improvement in symptoms and/or a slowing of the rate of deterioration of mental function.

As a general rule, anticholinesterase drugs should be used with caution in:
- heart rhythm abnormalities (particularly when the heart rate is low)
- asthma
- chronic obstructive pulmonary disease (COPD)
- epilepsy
- peptic ulcer

Although the individual cholinesterase drugs are listed below, in practice their side effects and potential interactions are similar. Most side effects are mild and short-lived, and can be reduced by taking the drugs with food.

DONEPEZIL

Main potential side effects
- headache
- difficulty in sleeping (insomnia)
- muscle cramps
- fatigue
- disturbances of the gut such as diarrhoea, constipation, nausea, vomiting, abdominal pain or stomach ulcer

- abnormal heart rhythm
- dizziness
- mood changes
- loss of appetite
- disturbances of liver function

How can this medicine affect other medicines?

The breakdown of donepezil may be inhibited by the following medicines, resulting in increased effects:

- erythromycin
- fluoxetine
- ketoconazole
- quinidine
- itraconazole

When taken together with the following medicines, the breakdown of donepezil may be accelerated, resulting in decreased effects:

- carbamazepine
- phenytoin
- rifampicin
- alcohol

Brand name

Aricept®

GALANTAMINE

Main potential side effects

- headache
- confusion
- fatigue
- disturbances of the gut such as diarrhoea, constipation, nausea, vomiting or abdominal pain

- weight loss
- indigestion
- very slow heart rate
- dizziness
- loss of appetite
- inflammation of the lining of the nose (rhinitis), causing a blocked or runny nose

This medicine may cause weight loss. Body weight should be regularly monitored in people taking it. Reminyl 12mg tablets contain the colouring E110, which may cause allergic reactions. Reminyl tablets contain lactose monohydrate as an inactive ingredient. This means that they are not suitable to be taken by people with rare hereditary problems of galactose intolerance, the Lapp lactase deficiency or glucose-galactose malabsorption. Reminyl oral solution does not contain lactose but does contain methyl and propyl parahydroxybenzoates, which can sometimes cause (possibly delayed) allergic reactions.

How can this medicine affect other medicines?
Galantamine has the potential to slow down the heart rate. If it is taken with other medicines that have this effect, such as digoxin and beta blockers, this effect may be enhanced.

Galantamine will antagonise the effects of medicines which act by blocking or decreasing the actions of acetylcholine (anticholinergic medicines), and so should not be taken with them. These medicines include hyoscine, atropine, benzhexol, procyclidine, ipratropium, oxitropium and oxybutinin.

Galantamine should not be taken with other medicines which increase the activity of acetylcholine, such as donepezil, rivastigmine, neostigmine, distigmine and pyridostigmine.

The blood levels of galantamine may be increased when taken with the following medicines:

- the SSRI antidepressants paroxetine, fluoxetine and fluvoxamine

- erythromycin
- quinidine
- ketoconazole
- ritonavir

Brand names

Reminyl oral solution®
Reminyl tablets®

RIVASTIGMINE

Main potential side effects

- headache
- rash
- difficulty in sleeping, or excessive sleepiness
- depression
- confusion
- shaking, usually of the hands
- sweating
- agitation
- indigestion
- ulceration of the stomach or intestine
- false perceptions of things that are not really there (hallucinations)
- dizziness
- seizures
- chest pain (angina)
- weakness or loss of strength
- decreased appetite and weight loss
- fainting
- disturbances of the gut such as nausea, vomiting, diarrhoea or abdominal pain

Brand name

Exelon®

MEMANTINE

How does it work?

This medicine contains the active ingredient memantine hydrochloride, which is a type of medicine called an NMDA-receptor antagonist. It is used for treating Alzheimer's disease. One of the ways in which memory loss and dementia in Alzheimer's disease are thought to occur is because of excessive activity of a neurotransmitter called glutamate.

Glutamate acts on nerve cell receptors called NMDA receptors. Glutamate can damage the nerve cells by excessively stimulating the NMDA receptors. Memantine works by blocking the NMDA receptors in the brain, and hence the excessive activity of glutamate. Memantine is licensed to treat moderately severe to severe Alzheimer's disease.

Use with caution in

- epilepsy
- heart failure
- decreased kidney function
- people who have recently had a heart attack
- uncontrolled high blood pressure (hypertension)

Main potential side effects

- headache
- tiredness
- vomiting
- confusion
- increased tension in the muscles
- false perceptions of things that are not really there (hallucinations)
- dizziness
- anxiety
- increased sex drive (libido)
- inflammation of the urinary bladder, commonly caused by infection (cystitis)

How can this medicine affect other medicines?

Memantine may alter the effects of the following medicines, and if you are taking any of these in combination with memantine your doctor may need to alter their doses:

- levodopa and other similar drugs for Parkinson's disease
- anticholinergic medicines for movement disorders such as Parkinson's disease (e.g. procyclidine) or intestinal cramps (e.g. atropine)
- antipsychotic medicines
- drugs for muscle spasm such as dantrolene and baclofen
- anti-ulcer drugs such as cimetidine and ranitidine

Brand name
Ebixa®

Appendix C

Useful contacts and addresses

Alzheimer's Society

The Alzheimer's Society is the leading dementia charity in England, Wales and Northern Ireland. The equivalent organisation in Scotland is Alzheimer's Scotland. Both provide services and campaign actively to help people with dementia and their families and carers.

Alzheimer's Society
Gordon House
10 Greencoat Place
London SW1P 1PH
Tel: 020 7306 0606
Fax: 020 7306 0808

Helpline
The national helpline can provide information, support, advice and referrals to other appropriate organisations. It is open from 8.30 a.m. to 6.30 p.m. from Monday to Friday.
Tel: 0845 300 0336

Alzheimer Scotland
22 Drumsheugh Gardens
Edinburgh
EH3 7RN
Tel: 0131 243 1453
Fax: 0131 243 1450
Helpline: 0808 808 3000 (24 hours)
www.alzscot.org

Age Concern

Age Concern aims to provide support to all people over 50 in the UK, to help ensure that they get the most from life. They provide essential services such as day care and information, and work to influence public opinion and government policy about older people.

Age Concern England
Astral House
1268 London Road
London SW16 4ER
Tel: 020 8765 7200
Fax: 020 8765 7240
www.ageconcern.org.uk

Age Concern Scotland
113 Rose Street
Edinburgh EH2 3DT
Tel: 0131 220 3345
Fax: 0131 220 2779
www.ageconcernscotland.org.uk

Age Concern Cymru
4th Floor
1 Cathedral Road
Cardiff CF11 9SD
Tel: 029 2037 1566
Fax: 029 2039 9562
www.accymru.org.uk

Age Concern Northern Ireland
3 Lower Crescent
Belfast BT7 1NR
Tel: 0289 024 5729
Fax: 0289 023 5497
www.ageconcernni.org

Pick's Disease Support Group

8 Brooksby Close
Oadby
Leicester
LE2 5AB
Tel: 0116 271 1414
Fax: 0870 706 0958
www.pdsg.org.uk